THE STATE OF THE WORLD'S CHILDREN
1995

Oxford University Press, Walton Street,
Oxford, OX2 6DP, Oxfordshire, U.K.
Oxford, New York, Toronto, Delhi, Bombay,
Calcutta, Madras, Karachi, Kuala Lumpur,
Singapore, Hong Kong, Tokyo, Nairobi,
Dar-es-Salaam, Cape Town, Melbourne,
Auckland and associated companies in
Berlin and Ibadan.

Oxford is a trade mark of Oxford University
Press.
Published in the United States by
Oxford University Press, New York.

Any part of The State of the World's Children
may be freely reproduced with the
appropriate acknowledgement.

British Library Cataloguing in
Publication Data
The state of the world's children 1995
1. Children – Care and hygiene
613' 0432 RJ101
ISBN 0-19-262642-6

ISSN 0265-718X

The Library of Congress has catalogued this
serial publication as follows:
The state of the world's children – Oxford and
New York: Oxford University Press for UNICEF
v.; ill.; 20cm. Annual. Began publication in
1980.
1. Children - Developing countries - Periodicals.
2. Children - Care and hygiene - Developing
countries - Periodicals. I. UNICEF.
HQ 792.2.S73 83-647550 362.7' 1'091724

UNICEF, UNICEF House, 3 U.N. Plaza,
New York, N.Y. 10017, U.S.A.
UNICEF, Palais des Nations, CH. 1211,
Geneva 10, Switzerland.

Cover photo: Claude Sauvageot
Design: Richard Gillingwater, Abingdon, U.K.
Typesetting: Duncan Carr, Wallingford, U.K.
Charts: Stephen Hawkins, Oxford, U.K.
Printing: Burgess (Abingdon) Ltd., U.K.

Edited and produced for UNICEF and
Oxford University Press by P & L Adamson,
18 Observatory Close, Benson, Wallingford,
Oxon OX10 6NU, U.K.
tel 0491-838431, fax 0491-825426

THE STATE OF THE WORLD'S CHILDREN 1995

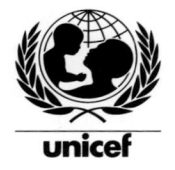

James P. Grant
Executive Director of the
United Nations Children's Fund

PUBLISHED FOR UNICEF

Oxford University Press

CONTENTS

The State of the World's Children 1995

1 *World of difference*

The tragedy of Rwanda's children is the latest in a series of such disasters. More quietly, the economic marginalization of even larger numbers of families is also depriving millions of children of the right to develop normally in mind and body. Both of these issues - increasing instability and increasing economic exclusion - will be on the agenda of the 1995 World Summit for Social Development in Copenhagen. The Summit is expected to draw up a new strategy for international development. But it will not resolve the emerging crisis in human security unless it gives priority to protecting and investing in the physical, mental, and emotional development of the world's children.

page 1

2 *Promise and progress*

Following the 1990 World Summit for Children, an important beginning has been made in this direction. The Summit set specific and measurable goals - to be achieved by the year 2000 - for the protection of the health and development of the world's children. It was subsequently agreed that a set of intermediate goals should be achieved by the end of 1995.

Chapter 2 looks at the practical progress that has been made - and finds that a majority of the goals set for 1995 are likely to be met by a majority of the developing nations. These achievements are an important contribution to the Copenhagen Summit - and to the task of translating words into deeds.

page 12

3 *Words into deeds*

The strategies behind the achievements recorded in chapter 2 have included: the breaking down of overall aims into 'doable' propositions; the securing of political support; the mobilization of new communications capacities; the deployment of United Nations expertise; and the close monitoring of progress. The task facing the World Summit for Social Development is to break down the broader challenges of today's development consensus into doable propositions.

page 35

4 *Pain now, gain later*

More fundamental change is also necessary. In particular, the problems of discrimination, landlessness and unemployment must be addressed. But the way forward is obstructed by political and economic vested interests, and by the 'pain now, gain later' nature of many of the necessary policies.

page 43

5 *Unfinished business of the 20th century*

The effort to achieve social development goals is part of a historic struggle to overcome such vested interests and to restructure societies in the interests of the many rather than the few. Completing this revolution is the unfinished business of the 20th century.

page 52

Statistical tables

All-country statistical tables for basic indicators, nutrition, health, education, population, economic progress, and the situation of women, plus regional summaries, and basic indicators for less populous countries.

page 63

Text figures

Fig. 1	Total debt as a percentage of GNP, 1980-1992	*page 7*
Fig. 2	United Nations projections of world population growth - low, medium, and high variants	*page 9*
Fig. 3	Estimated impact of iodine deficiency worldwide	*page 14*
Fig. 4	Number of developing countries where the mid-decade goal of iodizing at least 95% of salt in countries affected by iodine deficiency disorders is likely to be met	*page 16*
Fig. 5	Number of developing countries where the mid-decade goal of reducing 1990 child malnutrition by 20% is likely to be met	*page 17*
Fig. 6	Estimated impact of vitamin A deficiency on under-fives in the developing world	*page 18*
Fig. 7	Number of developing countries where the mid-decade goal of eliminating vitamin A deficiency in affected countries is likely to be met	*page 19*
Fig. 8	Percentage of all women and of pregnant women suffering from iron deficiency anaemia	*page 20*
Fig. 9	Percentage of the developing world's under-ones protected against five of the major vaccine-preventable diseases	*page 21*
Fig. 10	Number of developing countries where the mid-decade goal of reaching or maintaining an 80% immunization level is likely to be met	*page 21*
Fig. 11	Changes in the estimated numbers of polio cases in the developing world compared with changes in polio immunization	*page 23*
Fig. 12	Changes in under-five deaths from measles in the developing world compared with changes in measles immunization	*page 25*
Fig. 13	Tetanus immunization of pregnant women in the developing world compared with changes in infant deaths from tetanus	*page 27*
Fig. 14	Percentage of diarrhoea bouts in under-fives treated with oral rehydration in the developing world	*page 28*
Fig. 15	Number of developing countries where the mid-decade goal of ensuring 80% ORT use for diarrhoeal disease is likely to be met	*page 28*
Fig. 16	Percentage of villages with endemic dracunculiasis having one or more control interventions at the end of 1993	*page 29*
Fig. 17	Percentage of 6-11-year-olds enrolled in school	*page 31*
Fig. 18	Number of developing countries where the mid-decade goal of reducing the primary education shortfall by one third is likely to be met	*page 31*
Fig. 19	Number of developing countries where the mid-decade goal of reducing the safe water shortfall by one quarter is likely to be met	*page 33*
Fig. 20	Official development assistance from the 21 member nations of the OECD Development Assistance Committee	*page 34*
Fig. 21	Numbers and percentage of population below the poverty line in developing countries, 1985 and 1990	*page 44*
Fig. 22	Social and economic indicators for the Indian state of Kerala, compared with India as a whole	*page 49*
Fig. 23	Progress in life expectancy, under-five mortality, total fertility rate, and net primary school enrolment, developing world, 1960-1990	*page 55*

Panels

1 **Population:**
the Cairo consensus
page 4

2 **The year 2050:**
Vision 1
page 6

3 **The year 2050:**
Vision 2
page 8

4 **Social goals:**
1995 and 2000
page 10

5 **AIDS:**
the children's tragedy
page 22

6 **Mexico:**
30,000 saved since 1990
page 24

7 **The greatest abuse:**
violence against women
page 26

8 **Viet Nam:**
using the Convention
page 30

9 **Real aid:**
for real development
page 32

10 **The PPE spiral:**
and the new security crisis
page 58

Words into deeds

The 1990 World Summit for Children agreed on a series of specific goals for improving the lives of children - including measurable progress against malnutrition, preventable disease, and illiteracy.

Four years later, what practical progress has been made?

In sum, the answer is that more than 100 of the developing nations, with over 90% of the developing world's children, are making significant progress towards the goals. And on present trends, a majority of the targets set for 1995 are expected to be met by a majority of the developing nations.

Malnutrition has been reduced; immunization levels are generally being maintained or increased; measles deaths are down by 80% compared to pre-immunization levels; large areas of the developing world have become free of polio; iodine deficiency disorders and vitamin A deficiency are being overcome; the use of oral rehydration therapy (ORT) is rising (preventing more than a million child deaths a year); guinea worm disease has been reduced by some 90% and complete eradication is in sight; thousands of hospitals are actively supporting breastfeeding; progress in primary education is being resumed; and the Convention on the Rights of the Child has become the most widely and rapidly ratified convention in history.

Such progress means that approximately 2.5 million fewer children will die in 1996 than in 1990. It also means that tens of millions will be spared the insidious sabotage wrought on their development by malnutrition. And it means that at least three quarters of a million fewer children each year will be disabled, blinded, crippled, or mentally retarded.

For the first time, therefore, a series of internationally agreed social development goals is being made good on a significant scale in a majority of countries.

Chapter 2 of this year's State of the World's Children *report provides a more detailed summary of the progress being made towards the goals adopted at the 1990 World Summit for Children.*

World of difference

SUMMARY: The tragedy of Rwanda's children is the latest in what appears to be an increasingly frequent sequence of such disasters. More quietly, the economic marginalization of even larger numbers of families is also casting a long shadow over the future of nations by depriving millions of children of the right to develop normally in mind and body. The mutually reinforcing relationship between these two forces - increasing economic exclusion and increasing social disintegration - is at the core of a new generation of threats to human security.

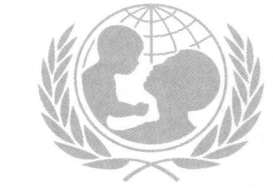

These threats will be the main issue facing the World Summit for Social Development which will convene in Copenhagen in March of 1995. The Summit should be the beginning of an attempt to implement the consensus on development issues that has begun to emerge in the 1990s. International action for development may be entering a new and more urgent phase: the relationships between poverty, population growth, environmental deterioration, rising aspirations, and social dislocation, are transforming the struggle against poverty from being a timeless issue of concern mainly to the poor into a race against time in which all nations have a stake.

The world will not solve these problems unless it puts protecting and investing in children at the centre of any new development strategy. Following the 1990 World Summit for Children, an important beginning has been made in this direction. A mid-1994 review suggests that a majority of the social development goals set for the middle of this decade will be achieved by a majority of the developing countries. These achievements - and the strategies which have brought them about - are an important contribution to the Copenhagen Summit: for the real challenge facing the World Summit for Social Development is not the further articulation of what should be done but the finding of ways and means to begin translating words into deeds.

The centrepiece of this year's *State of the World's Children* report is an account of what is being achieved - in practice - following the specific promises that were made by governments at the 1990 World Summit for Children.

But any review of what is happening to children in the world of 1994 must begin on a note of anger and sadness at the suffering endured by the children of Rwanda - suffering of a scale and a severity that the human mind cannot adequately encompass.

It is in the tradition of this annual report to stand back from such particular events in order to take a broader

At one time, wars were fought between armies; but in the wars of the last decade far more children than soldiers have been killed and disabled.

view of the forces affecting the lives of children in the late 20th century. But even that broader view must recognize that the tragedy of Rwanda is not an isolated occurrence. It is, rather, the latest and worst in what appears to be an increasingly frequent series of catastrophes for children, whether in Mozambique or Angola, Somalia or the Sudan, Afghanistan or Cambodia, Haiti or Bosnia.

All of these conflicts, made the more devastating by weapons exported from the industrialized nations, have brought not only short-term suffering to millions of families but long-term consequences for the development of people and of nations. What kind of adults will they be, these millions of children who have been traumatized by mass violence, who have been denied the opportunity to develop normally in mind and body, who have been deprived of homes and parents, of family and community, of identity and security, of schooling and stability? What scars will they carry forward into their own adult lives, and what kind of contribution will they be making to their societies in 15 or 20 years from now?

The nature of such conflicts is changing. At one time, wars were fought between armies; but in the wars of the last decade far more children than soldiers have been killed and disabled. Over that period, approximately 2 million children have died in wars, between 4 and 5 million have been physically disabled, more than 5 million have been forced into refugee camps, and more than 12 million have been left homeless.

These are statistics of shame. And they cast a long shadow over future generations and their struggle for stability and social cohesion.

Marginalization

But the broader view must also recognize that armed conflict is not the only force which is affecting the normal development of millions of children in the 1990s. More quietly, the continued economic and social marginalization of the poorest nations, and of the poorest communities within nations, is depriving far larger numbers of children of the kind of childhood which would enable them to become part of tomorrow's solutions rather than tomorrow's problems.

In the last 10 years, in particular, falling commodity prices, rising military expenditures, poor returns on investment, the debt crisis, and structural adjustment programmes, have reduced the real incomes of approximately 800 million people in some 40 developing countries. In Latin America, the fall in incomes has been as much as 20%. In sub-Saharan Africa, it has often been much more. At the same time, cuts in essential social services have meant health centres without drugs and doctors, schools without books and teachers, family planning clinics without staff and supplies.

For many millions of families in the poorest villages and urban slums of the developing world, the daily consequence of these economic forces, over which they have no control, is that they are unable to put enough food on the table, unable to maintain a home fit to live in, unable to dress and present themselves decently, unable to protect health and strength, unable to keep their children in school.

Through such processes, millions have become destitute and desperate. And when the destitute and the desperate are increasingly young, uprooted, urbanized, knowing far more about the world than their parents did and expecting far more from it, then the almost inevitable result is an increase in social disintegration, ethnic tensions, and political turbulence. Inevitable, also, is the rise of crime, violence, alcoholism, and drug abuse, by which a minority of the aggrieved and the discarded have always sought to console themselves.

Through all complexity and regional diversity, a pattern of economic marginalization can increasingly be discerned. Its identifying motif is the steady marginalization of the poorest nations and of the poorest people within nations. Internationally, the poorest 40 or 50 countries have seen their share of world income decline to the point where a fifth of the world's people now share less than 1.5% of world income.[1] Within individual nations, developing or industrialized, the poorest sections of the community are also being increasingly marginalized: in the 44 developing nations and 20 industrialized countries for which figures are available, the poorest fifth now share, on average, little more than 5% of national income, while the richest fifth claim between 40% and 60%.[2]

This tendency is not confined to the developing world: in many industrialized nations a significant fraction of the population is also being excluded from social and economic progress. During the decade of the 1980s, for example, 4 million more American children fell below the official poverty line even as average incomes rose and the economy as a whole grew by 25%.[3] Similarly, in the United Kingdom, the proportion of the employed who earn less than half the average national income has doubled in the last three decades.[4]

An underclass is therefore being created, undereducated and unskilled, standing beneath the broken bottom rungs of social and economic progress, victims of past poverty, of falling real wages, and of the fraying of social safety nets in the 1980s.

Alongside the more visible tragedies of violent conflict or sudden catastrophe, this quieter process of economic marginalization is also affecting many millions of children in the world of 1994, increasing the likelihood that they will fail to grow to their physical and mental potential, fail to complete school, fail to find work, and fail to become well-adjusted, economically productive, and socially responsible adults.

These two different kinds of threat - increasing tension and increasing exclusion - are not separate issues. It may be that, as one historian has written, *"In all epochs men of one creed, class, race or state have tended to despise, hate and fear men of alien identities;"*[5] but it is also the case that such tendencies are more likely to be kept within bounds by social and economic progress, by a reasonably equitable distribution of its benefits, and by the evolution of stable democracies, laws and institutions. No circumstances can wash the blood from the individual hands that have committed this year's crimes in Bosnia or Rwanda, but it would be a mistake to conclude that the root of such atrocities is ethnic and tribal hatred alone.

World Summit

The mutually reinforcing relationship between these two forces - increasing economic exclusion and increasing social disintegration - is the mainspring of a new generation of threats to human security. These threats will be the main issue facing the World Summit for Social Development, which will bring the majority of the world's political leaders to Copenhagen during March of 1995.

Setting out the political background to the Summit, the Secretary-General of the United Nations, Boutros Boutros-Ghali, has argued that direct aggression by one country against another has now become rare, and that the traditional concept of security - the territorial security of states that was the original purpose of the United Nations - has been largely achieved.[6] But within those states, there is today a *"new crisis in human security."* And its most obvious manifestations are increasing internal conflicts, mass migration to marginal lands and urban slums, frustrated aspirations, rising social tensions, and the disaffection of large numbers of people from their societies, their value systems, their governments, and their institutions. Internationally, the new threats include the increase in the number of failed states and in the need for international intervention, the mass migration of refugees within and between countries, the rise in international drug trafficking and organized crime,

An underclass is being created, undereducated and unskilled, standing beneath the broken bottom rungs of social and economic progress.

Panel 1

Population: the Cairo consensus

"Empowerment of individual women, opening a wider range of choice for both women and men, ... may be the key to social development, including the resolution of population problems, in the rest of the century and beyond."

Dr. Nafis Sadik
Executive Director, United Nations Population Fund

Media coverage of the 1994 International Conference on Population and Development focused on passionate disputes about abortion and sex education. But the remarkable feature of the Cairo Conference was the equally passionate agreement that the population issue revolves around women having greater control of their own lives, including their own fertility. In particular, there was wide agreement on the need to reduce the levels of abortion and maternal mortality, to extend reproductive health services to women in all communities, to raise levels of female education, and to accelerate progress towards gender equality.

An estimated half a million women die each year - and many times that number suffer injury and disability - from the complications of pregnancy and giving birth (including unsafe abortions). About a third of those pregnancies are unplanned and unwanted, and most fall into high-risk categories. Empowering women to decide whether and when to become pregnant, through greater equality in decision-making and high-quality family planning services, could reduce this dreadful toll. It could prevent the undermining of long-term health caused by too many births too close together; it could allow girls to mature physically and emotionally, and to complete their education, before they become mothers; and it could allow women more time to pursue other opportunities - and for the rest and recreation that is today almost entirely denied to millions of women in the developing world.

In an ideal world, the spread of family planning and the slowing down of population growth would therefore be a by-product of, rather than the motivation for, the meeting of women's basic rights and needs.

The Cairo Conference drew on the last 20 years of study and experience to show that the principal forces behind falling fertility are: rising levels of education, particularly for girls; lower child death rates (enabling parents to have confidence that their children will survive); increasing economic security; progress towards gender equality (helping to reduce son preference and offering women choices beyond unbroken years of child-bearing); and the widespread availability of family planning information and services.

All of these determinants of population growth are responses to the basic needs and rights of individuals, and all would cry out to be achieved even if there were no such thing as a population problem. In this sense also, a continued rapid fall in the rate of world population growth would be a by-product of, rather than a motivation for, such changes.

But if extra incentive is needed, then it is now clear that taking action on all of these fronts would fundamentally alter the future pattern of population growth. The present population of the world is approximately 5.6 billion. The United Nations 'medium variant' projection for world population in the year 2050 is approximately 10 billion. The high projection is 12.5 billion. No single intervention short of catastrophe can make a fundamental difference to those figures. But the Cairo Conference concluded that a comprehensive approach - combining progress in child health and survival, progress in education, progress towards gender equality, and the universal availability of family planning - could keep world population to less than 10 billion by the middle of the next century.

The differences between these projected figures could represent the difference between success and failure in effecting the transition to a sustainable future. □

the continued legal and illegal trade in weapons, and the threat to the biosphere caused by overconsumption and overpollution.

All of these represent new and different threats to human security, and they require a new and different response from the international community and from the United Nations.

The purpose of the Copenhagen Summit is to try to find such a response. And its starting-point must be that no answer can be adequate if it does not include a commitment to a new kind of international development effort that will do a better job of protecting the growing minds and bodies of children, that will acknowledge the rights and needs of women, and that will generate the kind of job-creating and environmentally sustainable economic growth which includes rather than excludes the poorest nations and the poorest people. As Boutros Boutros-Ghali has said: *"A shared commitment to social progress is the answer to shared threats of poverty, unemployment, and social disintegration ... It is time to shift from providing security through arms, to ensuring security through development."*[7]

The challenge for Copenhagen

The coming together of a majority of the world's heads of state to discuss the issues of poverty, unemployment, and social exclusion is unprecedented. And the very fact of the Copenhagen Summit is an indication of two important new developments. The first is a rising political awareness of new threats to human security - and of the fact that the international community must begin to address the causes if it is not to be overwhelmed by the symptoms. The second is a narrowing of many of the fundamental divides of recent years and its replacement by a new level of consensus. As the Chairman of the Preparatory Committee for the World Summit for Social Development, Juan Somavia, has observed: *"Ten years ago this Summit would have been impossible. It would have been an ideological debate about economic and social systems."*[8]

As these fundamental differences in approach have been beaten into shallower relief, a more particular consensus on development issues has also begun to emerge. It is the outcome of the experience, trials, and errors, of more than 40 years of conscious development efforts. It is the outcome of many reports and analyses from United Nations agencies and non-governmental organizations. It is the outcome of the work of the many distinguished commissions which have inquired into these issues in recent years - the Brandt Commission, the Brundtland Commission, the Palme Commission, and the South Commission. It is the outcome of a series of major summit meetings, including the World Summit for Children in 1990 and the Earth Summit in 1992. And it is the outcome of the recent Cairo International Conference on Population and Development which has set out a clear and vital message to the world on the complex reciprocal relationships between the needs and rights of women, changes in fertility, and progress towards sustainable development (panel 1).

More than at any other time in the 50-year history of the United Nations, it can therefore be said that there is today a broad measure of agreement on many of the most basic problems of development and their most likely solutions.

That consensus has been set out many times, including in last year's *State of the World's Children* report, and need not be reiterated here. Suffice it to say that, with varying combinations of emphases, there is today a considerable agreement that the way forward lies along the path of democratic politics and market-friendly economics; of government action to ensure that growth benefits the many and not just the few; of meeting human needs and investing in human capacities through better health, nutrition, and education; of the restructuring of government expenditures and aid programmes in favour of basic social services and employment opportunities

There is today a broad measure of agreement on many of the most basic problems of development and their most likely solutions.

Panel 2

The year 2050 Vision 1

The panels on this page and overleaf set out two alternative visions of the world in the middle of the 21st century. They illustrate why the struggle against world poverty is now being transformed into a race against time.

No new international effort has been made to overcome the worst of poverty and underdevelopment. Economic marginalization has been allowed to continue and the inequalities of the 20th century have deepened. Continued malnutrition and poor health care have left child death rates at relatively high levels for large numbers of people. Little has been done to achieve equality between the sexes. More than 100 million primary school age children, two thirds of them girls, are not in school. Secondary school remains the preserve of a minority, and average age at marriage has risen only marginally. Many of the poor have therefore continued to have large families to compensate for high death rates, to ensure surviving sons, and to try to insure themselves against destitution. Women still do not have the power to control their own fertility, and many families who want fewer children still do not have access to high-quality family planning.

As the year 2050 approaches, total world population is nearing the 12 billion mark and continuing to rise. The population of Africa has trebled to approximately 2 billion people. Vastly greater numbers of the poor are working ever more marginal lands. The cutting of forests and the erosion of hillsides have accelerated, resulting in scarcity of food and fuel. Rivers, dams and irrigation systems are silting up, much of the best farm land has become saline or waterlogged, and lowland areas are subject to increasingly frequent and disastrous floods. Millions have migrated to urban slums, where poverty, overcrowding, and poor sanitation make life almost unbearable and where the chief form of entertainment involves sophisticated communications technologies constantly parading the images of wealth before the realities of poverty. Traditional community structures and values have long since broken down, and a significant proportion of the desperate have turned to crime, or are seeking relief in alcohol and drugs.

Social divisions and old ethnic tensions have increased and, in the resulting political turmoil, democracies have faltered, leaving the way open for demagogues and dictators who have grown like weeds in such soil. More resources are being devoted to the military, and to the security forces on whom they depend.

Increasing civil and international conflicts are providing a ready market for an arms trade that has been allowed to continue unabated. Many civil wars have degenerated into causeless struggles for power and territory. Refugee problems have multiplied. Internal and international migration pressures have increased. Acts of international terrorism have become more common, committed both by increasing numbers of criminal groups and by the many organizations motivated by frustration and deeply felt injustice. Many airports have become unusable. Insurance costs have risen steeply. Travel and commerce are disrupted. Investment and tourism have declined. More than one hard-pressed dictator uses the lightning-rod of foreign adventurism to distract attention from domestic problems. The number of failed states increases. International intervention becomes more common in an attempt to cope with instability, and limited global resources are diverted not to development but to peace-keeping and emergencies.

Meanwhile, the established industrialized nations continue to consume and pollute, and have been joined by several of the most populous Asian and Latin American nations whose energy consumption and emissions of carbon dioxide and other pollutants have by now become considerably greater than those of the old industrialized world. □

for the poor; of ending the discrimination against women and girls that is so unacceptable in principle and so ruinous of development efforts in practice;* of reducing fertility through a comprehensive approach combining family planning information and services, lowered child death rates, improved levels of education, and the empowering of women to decide how many children to have and when; of rethinking unjust and unsustainable patterns of consumption and pollution in industrialized nations; of significant cuts in arms expenditures and an increase in the resources available for environmentally sustainable development; of a reorientation of economic assistance towards countries that spend less on military capacity and more on meeting the basic needs of the poorest; of debt cancellation and reduction for the least developed nations (fig. 1); of a new level of international effort to assist sub-Saharan Africa to resume its progress; and of a significant increase in the level and efficiency of investment in the developing world.[9]

Even the time-honoured debate about what is meant by development has given way to a broad agreement that has perhaps best been summed up by the Administrator of the United Nations Development Programme (UNDP):

"Sustainable human development is development that not only generates economic growth but distributes its benefits equitably; that regenerates the environment rather than destroying it; that empowers people rather than marginalizing them. It gives priority to the poor, enlarging their choices and opportunities, and provides for their participation in decisions affecting them. It is development that is pro-poor, pro-nature, pro-jobs, pro-democracy, pro-women, and pro-children."

Words and actions

But it is also fair to say that, in the past, recommendations and resolutions along the lines recommended by this consensus have not been followed by practical changes on the necessary scale.

Is there any reason to believe that the promises and resolutions that will undoubtedly be issued in Copenhagen will be any different?

This report will argue that the struggle against poverty is reaching a new and critical juncture, and that the prospects for a renewed international effort are improving. For as the recent International Conference on Population and Development in Cairo has made clear, there is today a new level of urgency about the development debate. Long treated as a 'timeless' issue of urgent concern only to the poor themselves, the struggle against world poverty is now being transformed into a race against time in which all have a stake (panels 2 and 3).

After decades of relative inaction, this is a potentially dramatic transformation. And it has been brought about by fundamental shifts in the substructure of human affairs. First, massive increases in productive capacity in recent years have made it possible for the basic benefits of progress to be put at the disposal of all the world's people. Second, an equally dramatic increase in communications capacity has made it obvious to people everywhere that this is the case - that poverty and malnutrition and disease and illiteracy are no longer inevitable. Third, a fundamental change in the accepted ethic of social organization (discussed more fully in chapter 5) is bringing the needs, rights, and expectations of the individual to centre stage, raising expectations of both material progress and social justice for millions of people who in previous ages have been encouraged to believe that such rights appertained only to the few. As a result of all of these forces, the gap between reality and possibility, for hundreds of millions of people, has grown so wide as to be unsustainable. If democracies are to be sustained, if the conduct of human affairs is not to lapse into widespread social disintegration and political upheaval, then this gap must rapidly be closed: reality must keep

Fig. 1 Debt burden

Total debt as percentage of GNP, 1980 to 1992.

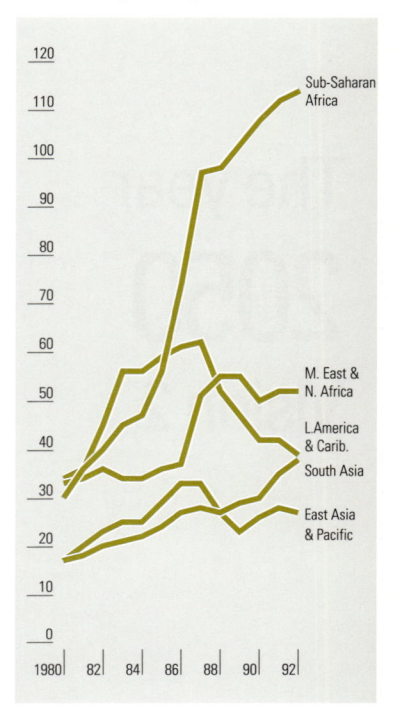

Source: *World Bank*, World debt tables 1993–94, *vol. 2, 1993.*

* This aspect of the consensus, already brought to the fore by the Cairo International Conference on Population and Development, will be further developed at the Fourth World Conference on Women, to be held in Beijing in September 1995.

Panel 3

The year 2050 Vision 2

The late 1990s and the early part of the 21st century saw a new international effort to overcome the worst of poverty and underdevelopment. Government expenditures and aid programmes were substantially restructured to invest in jobs and basic social services, including nutrition, health, and education. Governments also confronted the challenge of land tenure reform, training, and credit for small farmers, making major investments in environmentally sustainable increases in small-farm productivity. The surpluses generated have helped to create downstream employment, and most families have gained the means of meeting their basic needs. Governments also took a strong lead in promoting more rapid progress towards gender equality by giving special emphasis to female education, improved family planning services, technologies to lessen women's workloads, and equal opportunity legislation.

As a result of all of these measures, and of slowly rising incomes, child death rates have fallen steeply, average age at marriage has risen, opportunities for women have increased, having sons has become less important, and small families have become the norm. Population growth has peaked at about 8 billion people, and is set to decline.

Investments in small landholdings and new agricultural technologies have prevented worsening erosion and slowed the drift to the cities. As a result of slowly improving educational standards and increasing economic security, civilian governments have become established and various forms of participatory democracy have become normal. The benefits of growth are now being shared reasonably equitably, people feel less alienated from their institutions, and the voice of the poor is no longer ignored in the allocation of public resources.

States have drawn back from the brink of collapse, and domestic and international resources have been gradually shifted from military and peace-keeping budgets to investments in economic development, social progress, and environmental protection. The established industrialized nations have all reduced military spending, restricted arms sales, and invested more financial and human resources in working with developing nations to find the technologies that can meet the legitimate aspirations of their 7 billion people for a higher standard of living while preserving the integrity of local and global environments.

Meanwhile, both old and new industrialized nations are taking advantage of the changes mandated by the environmental crisis to search for a pattern of progress which will lead to greater human satisfaction and social cohesion.

The choice between these two futures must be made not in 50 years time but today.

More than two decades when the world could have been addressing these urgent problems have already been lost. Another lost decade will probably be decisive. As UNDP Administrator James Gustave Speth recently testified:

"Forces have been unleashed in recent years that could give us, early in the new century, very different courses. We could witness large areas of the world dissolving into ethnic violence, poverty, hunger, and social and environmental disintegration. Or we could all be the beneficiaries of tremendous vitality and innovation for the creation of a new, just, and sustainable international order.... But we must act now with determination and urgency. Everything that must be done should have been done yesterday. Tomorrow it will be more costly. Time is the most important variable in the equation of the future." *

* James Gustave Speth, Administrator, United Nations Development Programme, address to the Secretary's Open Forum, United States Department of State, Washington, D.C., 2 March 1994.

step with possibility, morality with capacity.

Add to these forces the momentum of population growth, and the increasing degradation of marginal rural environments and urban slums, and the inevitability of fundamental change - in one direction or another - becomes plain. By the middle of the next century, total world population could be 12 billion and rising or 8 billion and falling (fig. 2). The difference between these two figures is roughly the equivalent of the entire population of the developing world today. It could also represent a world of difference in another sense - the difference between success and failure in preventing ecological and social catastrophe.

Given the choice, every sane person would opt for the lower population figure. But as the Cairo Conference again made clear, population growth cannot be contained by family planning alone. Only a comprehensive approach - combining greater economic security, the empowering of women to decide if and when to have children, higher educational standards (particularly for girls), lower child death rates so that parents can have confidence that their children will survive, and the universal availability of high-quality family planning information and services - has a chance of achieving a world population as low as 8 billion by the middle of the next century (panel 1).

Slowing population growth therefore means meeting the legitimate needs of the individual, particularly the individual woman, and accelerating progress against some of the worst aspects of poverty, malnutrition, disease, illiteracy, and gender discrimination. Such progress has long been demanded on humanitarian grounds, and would cry out to be achieved even if there were no such thing as a population problem. But there is a population problem. And this, too, is now lending new urgency to old demands.

In other words, overcoming the 'old' problems of poverty, landlessness, unemployment, malnutrition, illiteracy, disease, and discrimination is a prerequisite of successfully managing the 'new' problems of population growth, environmental deterioration, frustrated aspirations, and social disintegration. And as the threat represented by the new problems grows, it increases the urgency of efforts to resolve the old problems of poverty and underdevelopment.

In the past, the international development effort has lacked any real urgency; there have been no deadlines attached, no imperative other than the humanitarian, no spur other than the nag of conscience, no consequences of failure other than for the poor themselves. All this is now changing. Development now has a deadline. And failure to meet it will bring consequences not just for the poor but for all. Implementing today's development consensus is therefore becoming not only a moral minimum for our civilization but a practical minimum for ensuring its survival.

Children at the centre

This, then, is the background to the World Summit for Social Development in Copenhagen. The outcome asked for by the Secretary-General of the United Nations is nothing less than a new international strategy for social development.

This year's *State of the World's Children* report seeks to make two particular contributions to the Copenhagen Summit.

The first can be quickly stated. It is UNICEF's belief that the time has now come to put the needs and the rights of children at the very centre of development strategy.

This argument is based neither on institutional vested interest nor on sentimentality about the young; it is based on the fact that childhood is the period when minds and bodies and personalities are being formed and during which even temporary deprivation is capable of inflicting lifelong damage and distortion on human development. It follows that, whether the threat be war and conflict or economic marginal-

Fig. 2 The 21st century

United Nations projections of world population growth – low, medium, and high variants (in billions).

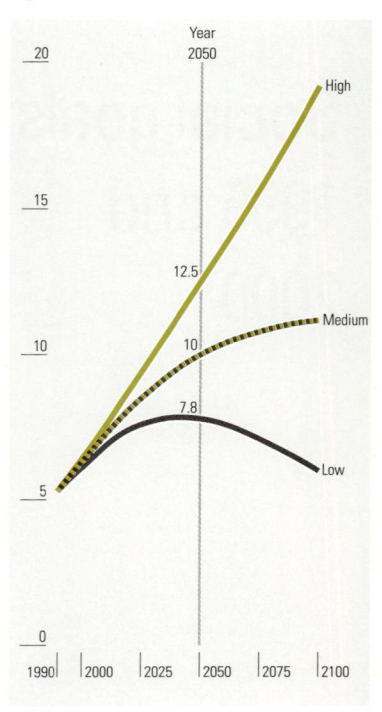

Source: *United Nations,* Long-range population projections: two centuries of population growth 1950–2010, *1992.*

Panel 4

Social goals: 1995 and 2000

Goals for the year 2000

The end-of-century goals, agreed to by almost all the world's governments following the 1990 World Summit for Children, may be summarized under ten priority points.

1. A one-third reduction in 1990 under-five death rates (or to 70 per 1,000 live births, whichever is less).

2. A halving of 1990 maternal mortality rates.

3. A halving of 1990 rates of malnutrition among the world's under-fives (to include the elimination of micronutrient deficiencies, support for breastfeeding by all maternity units, and a reduction in the incidence of low birth weight to less than 10%).

4. The achievement of 90% immunization among under-ones, the eradication of polio, the elimination of neonatal tetanus, a 90% reduction in measles cases, and a 95% reduction in measles deaths (compared to pre-immunization levels).

5. A halving of child deaths caused by diarrhoeal disease.

6. A one-third reduction in child deaths from acute respiratory infections.

7. Basic education for all children and completion of primary education by at least 80% - girls as well as boys.

8. Clean water and safe sanitation for all communities.

9. Acceptance in all countries of the Convention on the Rights of the Child, including improved protection for children in especially difficult circumstances.

10. Universal access to high-quality family planning information and services in order to prevent pregnancies that are too early, too closely spaced, too late, or too many.

Goals for 1995

The following are the goals that have been accepted by almost all nations for achievement by the end of 1995. Chapter 2 of The State of the World's Children 1995 *provides a mid-1994 progress report.*

1. Immunization against the six major vaccine-preventable diseases of childhood to reach at least 80% in all countries.

2. Neonatal tetanus to be virtually eliminated.

3. Measles deaths to be reduced by 95% and measles cases by 90% (compared with pre-immunization levels).

4. The elimination of polio in selected countries and regions (as a step towards worldwide elimination by the year 2000).

5. The ending of free or low-cost distribution of breastmilk substitutes in all maternity units and hospitals, and the achievement of 'baby-friendly' status for all major hospitals.

6. The achievement of 80% ORT use, as part of the effort to control diarrhoeal disease.

7. The virtual elimination of vitamin A deficiency.

8. The universal iodization of salt in countries affected by iodine deficiency disorders.

9. The virtual elimination of guinea worm disease.

10. The universal ratification of the Convention on the Rights of the Child.

ization, children should, as far as is humanly possible, be protected from the worst mistakes and malignancies of the adult world.

For this reason, the most constant strand of UNICEF advocacy over the years has been that the vital, vulnerable years of childhood should be given a first call on societies' concerns and capacities, and that this commitment should be maintained in good times and in bad. A child has only one chance to develop normally; and the protection of that one chance therefore demands the kind of commitment that will not be superseded by other priorities. There will always be something more immediate; there will never be anything more important.

With the Copenhagen Summit, the time has now come to see this issue of protecting the growing minds and bodies of children not as a matter of peripheral concern, to be dealt with by a little extra sympathy and charity, but as an issue which is integral to almost every other item on the Copenhagen agenda. It is an issue that can be simply stated - the world will not solve its major problems until it learns to do a better job of protecting and investing in the physical, mental, and emotional development of its children.

Summit for children

Since the World Summit for Children in 1990, it has been shown that putting children at the centre of development strategy is not only a logical proposition but also a practicable one. The world has the accumulated knowledge, the technologies, and the communications capacities to protect the normal growth and development of almost all children at relatively low cost. Reducing malnutrition, disease, and illiteracy are among the most achievable as well as the most fundamental of development's challenges.

Combined with the world's generally greater willingness to act in the interests of children, this means that action to protect the rising generation could and should be a leading edge of any new effort to accelerate progress against poverty, reduce the momentum of population growth, and pre-empt ecological and social crises.

As chapter 2 of this report will show, considerable practical and political momentum has already been mobilized behind this cause.

The 1990 World Summit for Children, the first of the major summit meetings on development issues in the 1990s, agreed on a series of measurable goals to be achieved by the end of the 1990s (panel 4). Those goals included major progress against malnutrition, preventable disease, and illiteracy among the children of the developing world. In total, 27 specific goals were agreed upon and eventually endorsed by over 150 Presidents and Prime Ministers.

Too often, the commitments made on such occasions are forgotten, their resolutions calling ever more feebly from within the locked rooms of the past, their promises echoing ever more emptily down the years. But the four years since the World Summit for Children have, in the main, been years of practical progress and measurable achievement. And with 18 months to go before mid-decade, a country-by-country review suggests that a majority of the goals set for the end of 1995 will be met by a majority of developing nations.

For the first time, therefore, a series of internationally agreed social development goals is being made good on a significant scale in a majority of countries. The story of these practical achievements - and of the strategies which have made them possible - occupies much of this year's *State of the World's Children* report and is UNICEF's principal contribution to the World Summit for Social Development.

2 *Promise and progress*

SUMMARY: At the 1990 World Summit for Children, the international community agreed on a series of specific and measurable goals for the protection of the lives, the health, and the normal growth and development of children. The goals included a halving of child malnutrition, control of the major childhood diseases, the eradication of polio and dracunculiasis, the elimination of micronutrient deficiencies, a halving of maternal mortality, the achievement of primary school education by at least 80% of children, the provision of clean water and safe sanitation to all communities, and the universal ratification of the Convention on the Rights of the Child. It was subsequently agreed that a set of intermediate goals should be achieved by the end of 1995.

This chapter looks at progress - in practice - since these promises were made. With 18 months to go before mid-decade, it finds that a majority of the goals set for 1995 are likely to be met by a majority of the developing nations.

On Monday, 1 October 1990, *The New York Times* carried a leading article on the World Summit for Children, which had been held on the previous day at the Headquarters of the United Nations. The Summit, bringing together representatives of over 150 governments including 71 heads of state, had formally adopted a series of goals for the year 2000, including a one-third reduction in child deaths, a halving of child malnutrition, immunization levels of 90%, control of the major childhood diseases, the eradication of polio, the elimination of micronutrient deficiencies, a halving of maternal mortality rates, primary school education for at least 80% of children, the provision of clean water and safe sanitation to all communities, and the universal ratification of the new Convention on the Rights of the Child.[10] It was subsequently agreed that a set of intermediate goals should be achieved by the end of 1995 (panel 4).

The New York Times commented: "The largest global Summit meeting in history pledged to do better by the world's children. Their promises were eloquent, their goals ambitious. But children cannot survive or thrive on promises. The world's leaders now have an obligation to find the resources and the political will necessary to translate hope into reality."[11]

Four years on, how much translation into reality has there been?

In sum, the answer is that more than 100 of the developing nations, with over 90% of the developing world's children, are making significant practical progress towards the goals that were set four years ago.

The measurement of this progress is plagued by imperfect statistics, and the achievements so far are vulnerable to unpredictable forces that can still bring major set-backs (the first nation in Africa to reach 80% immunization was the central African state of Rwanda). But it is clear that a majority of the goals set for 1995 will be met by a majority of the developing nations.

Malnutrition has been reduced; immunization levels are generally being maintained or increased; measles deaths are down by 80% compared to pre-immunization levels; large areas of the developing world, including all of the western hemisphere, have become free of polio; iodine deficiency disorders are being eliminated; vitamin A deficiency is in retreat; the use of oral rehydration therapy (ORT) is rising (preventing more than a million child deaths a year); guinea worm disease has been reduced by some 90% and complete eradication is in sight; thousands of major hospitals in developing and industrialized countries are now actively supporting breastfeeding; progress in primary education is being resumed; and the Convention on the Rights of the Child has become the most widely and rapidly ratified convention in history.

Such progress means that approximately 2.5 million fewer children will die in 1996 than in 1990. It also means that tens of millions will be spared the insidious sabotage wrought on their development by malnutrition. And it means that at least three quarters of a million fewer children each year will be disabled, blinded, crippled, or mentally retarded.

By and large, these achievements have not been extensively reported by national and international media. This may be because good news is more difficult to dramatize than bad, or it may be because progress of this kind is not an event that happens in a particular place and at a particular time, or it may be because these developments are of consequence chiefly to some of the poorest people and communities on earth. Whatever the reason, achievements and successes have gone virtually unnoticed amid the flow of conventional news coverage about the developing world, its corruptions and its conflicts, its droughts and its disasters, its famines and its failures.

But if these achievements have not made the nightly news, they have changed the daily lives of many millions of families in some of the world's poorest communities. And they are a suitable reply to those who believe that international gatherings produce only fine words and forgotten promises, that internationally agreed goals are only ever set and never met, that there is only disaster and failure to report from the developing world, or that the United Nations family of organizations is not effective in helping to make the world a better place.

Practical progress of this kind deserves to be more widely recognized both as an example of promises and commitments being made good and as an encouragement to the many hundreds of thousands of people and many thousands of organizations working at all levels and in almost all countries for the achievement of these goals.

The following pages therefore carry a 'translation into reality' report, failures as well as successes, for each of the main goals adopted at the 1990 World Summit for Children.

In 1990, some 18 million women became pregnant while suffering from a little-known dietary disorder. In almost all cases those women did not know, and still do not know, what that problem was.

In approximately 60,000 cases, the damage caused was so severe that the foetus died or the infant survived for only a few hours.

For approximately 120,000 of those women, pregnancy and delivery proceeded normally, and an apparently healthy baby was born. But in the first few months of life it became clear that all was not well. The infant was slow to respond to voices, and did not seem to recognize familiar faces. It was still possible to hope that there was nothing seriously wrong, but most of those mothers knew that a certain light that should have been there in the child's eyes was missing.

As these children reached the age of two, most had still not learned to walk. In some cases, the legs had never become fully extended, and the most the child could manage was a kind of awkward shuffle. Anxious comparisons were made with neighbours' children. Parents tried to reassure each other by noting that some children develop more slowly than others. But with each passing day, the differences seemed less ignorable. Other family members started to make comments. Whispers began in the community.

Sometime in 1992 or 1993, when most of those children had still not learned to stand or to say their first words, the parents' fears were first

Three quarters of a million fewer children each year will be disabled, blinded, crippled, or mentally retarded.

Iodine deficiency has condemned millions of children to cretinism, tens of millions to mental retardation, and hundreds of millions to subtler degrees of mental and physical impairment.

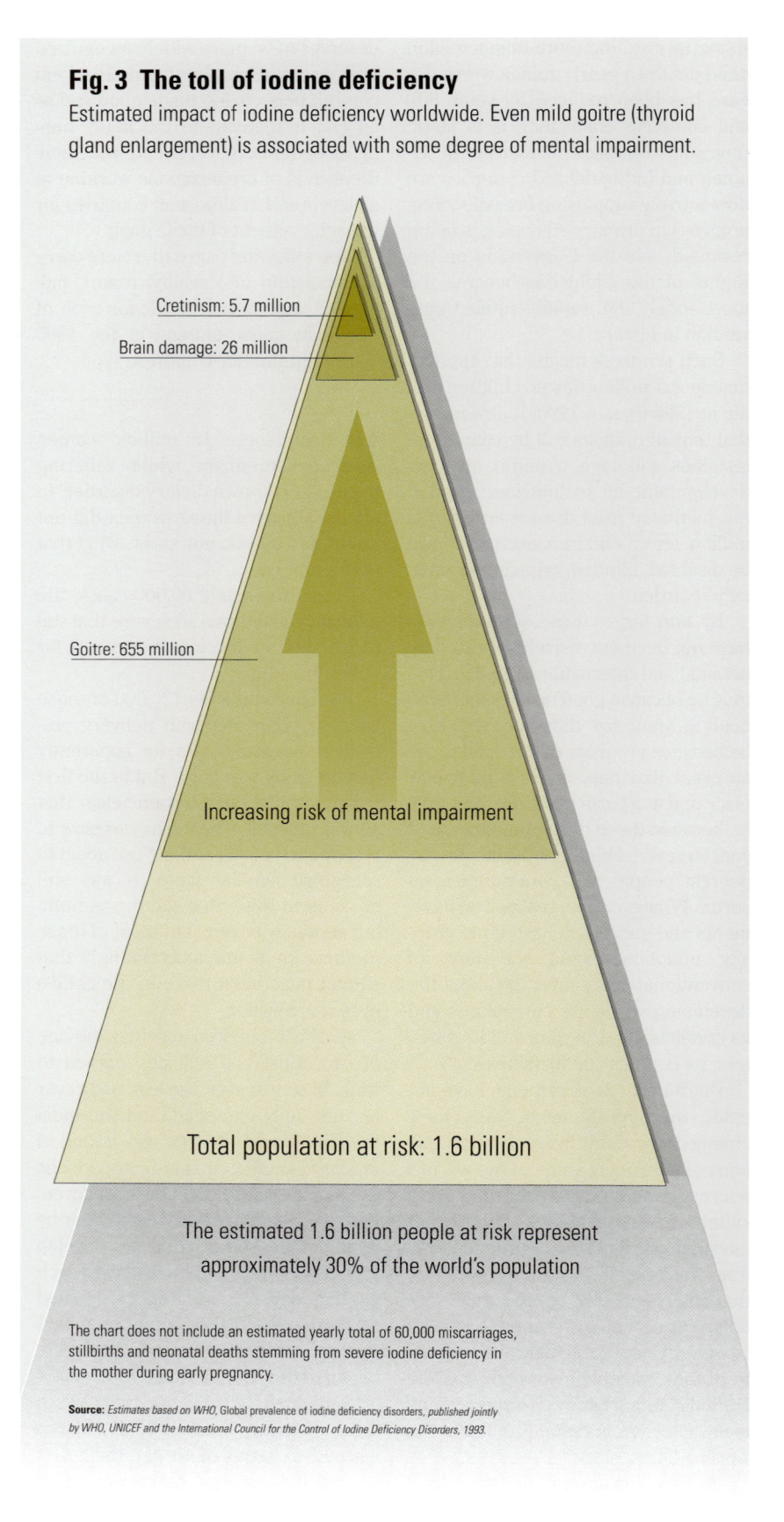

Fig. 3 The toll of iodine deficiency
Estimated impact of iodine deficiency worldwide. Even mild goitre (thyroid gland enlargement) is associated with some degree of mental impairment.

Cretinism: 5.7 million

Brain damage: 26 million

Goitre: 655 million

Increasing risk of mental impairment

Total population at risk: 1.6 billion

The estimated 1.6 billion people at risk represent approximately 30% of the world's population

The chart does not include an estimated yearly total of 60,000 miscarriages, stillbirths and neonatal deaths stemming from severe iodine deficiency in the mother during early pregnancy.

Source: *Estimates based on WHO,* Global prevalence of iodine deficiency disorders, *published jointly by WHO, UNICEF and the International Council for the Control of Iodine Deficiency Disorders, 1993.*

mentioned to a health worker or doctor. Many were told to come back in three months. Others were referred to clinics or hospitals for tests. Many waited long months for the results.

All were eventually informed that their children were severely and permanently retarded.

Very few ever learned the cause - that a dietary deficiency in pregnancy had damaged the development of their child's central nervous system.

Today, as those children reach their fourth and fifth birthdays, their parents know only that their sons or daughters were born as cretins, and will remain so for the rest of their lives.

There are no statistics on the feelings experienced in those 120,000 homes on hearing this news. No records to capture the unwarranted shame of acknowledging the problem to husbands, parents, in-laws, neighbours. No figures to measure the courage with which those 120,000 families, almost all of them desperately poor, have set about coping with the practical and economic difficulties that severe mental retardation brings in its long wake.

The story does not end there. In approximately 1 million more of those pregnancies, early childhood appeared to proceed quite normally. But today, as those 1 million children reach school age, many are being found to have poor eye-hand coordination; others have become partially deaf, or have developed a bad squint, or a speech impediment, or other neuromuscular disorders.

In another 5 million or so cases, the parents may never know that there is anything specifically wrong. But if measurements could be taken as those children embark on their first year at primary school, all of them, even the brightest, would be found to have significantly lowered IQs. And in the years to come, they will merge into the estimated total of 75 million young people in the world today whose mental and physical development, and capacity for education, are impaired by the same problem - arising either from their own diets in childhood or from the diets of their mothers before and during pregnancy. Eventually they will be added to the estimated total of 150 million adults whose diminished mental alertness and reduced physical aptitude mean that they are less able to meet their own and their families' needs.

Meanwhile, those most seriously affected, the 120,000 four- and five-year-old cretins born in 1990, will not be going to school at all. They will remain in the ranks of the dependent, eventually becoming part of the estimated 5.7 million people alive today who have been afflicted by cretinism from birth.[12]

Salt solution

The disorder which causes all of the above is the lack of minute amounts of iodine in the diet. The deficiency occurs mainly in hilly or flood-prone regions where iodine tends to be washed out of the soil, and the problems it gives rise to are collectively known as iodine deficiency disorders or IDD. In total, 1.6 billion people are at risk and 655 million suffer from goitre - the swelling of the thyroid gland at the throat which is the most obvious sign of IDD (fig. 3).

An inexpensive solution has been known for most of this century: iodine can be added to the one commodity that is consumed by all - common salt. That was how the problem was eradicated from most of the industrialized countries, led by Switzerland and the United States where edible salt supplies were iodized during the 1920s.

But in the developing world, the tragedy has been allowed to continue. And in the lifetime of most people reading this page, it has condemned millions of children to cretinism, tens of millions to mental retardation, and hundreds of millions to subtler degrees of mental and physical impairment.

The cost of salt iodization is approximately 5 US cents per person per year.

On 30 September 1990, the World Health Organization (WHO) and UNICEF confronted the world's politi-

Today, as those children reach their fourth and fifth birthdays, their parents know only that their sons or daughters were born as cretins.

Fig. 4 Meeting the mid-decade goals

Number of developing countries on track to achieve the mid-decade goal of iodizing at least 95% of salt in countries affected by iodine deficiency disorders.

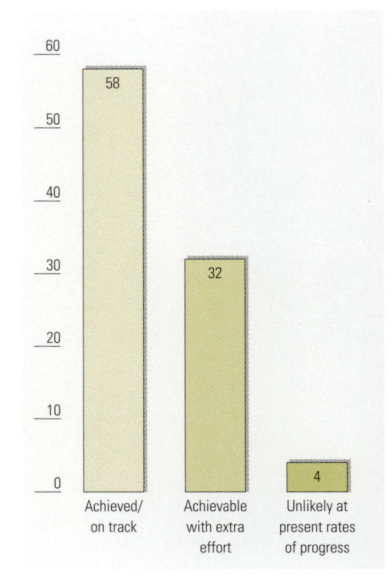

Achieved/on track	58
Achievable with extra effort	32
Unlikely at present rates of progress	4

Source: *Country assessments by UNICEF field staff, for 94 countries, September 1994.*

cal leaders with the challenge of salt iodization - along with several other equally powerful and equally inexpensive methods of preventing ill health, poor growth, and early death among many millions of the world's children.

The occasion was the World Summit for Children, held at the Headquarters of the United Nations in New York and attended by approximately half of the world's Presidents and Prime Ministers. On that day, the elimination of all new cases of iodine deficiency disorders by the year 2000 became one of 27 specific goals adopted by governments.[13]

To make that goal practicable, it was subsequently agreed that all countries would attempt the iodization of at least 95% of all salt supplies in each country by the end of 1995.

Just over four years later, what has been achieved?

Of the 94 countries with IDD problems, the great majority are now implementing national plans for the iodization of all salt and 58 are on track to achieve the goal of iodizing 95% of salt supplies by the end of 1995 (fig. 4). Those 58 countries are home to almost 60% of the developing world's children. Another 32 countries could achieve the 1995 goal with an accelerated effort.

In the Middle East and North Africa, 10 out of 17 nations will have iodized all salt within the next 12 months. In Asia, 7 out of 20 countries (including Bangladesh and India) are within a year of universal iodization. In India, the legislation requiring iodization has been passed, a monitoring system is being set up in every state, the necessary equipment is in place in every major salt-works, and over 50% of all salt is already iodized. In Central and South America, all nations with the possible exception of Haiti are likely to iodize all salt by the end of 1995 (although an acceleration of progress will be required in Colombia, Paraguay, and Peru). Bolivia and Ecuador, the two South American countries with the worst history of IDD, are very close to eliminating the problem. Remarkably, salt iodization is also being achieved in 28 of the 39 affected nations in sub-Saharan Africa where all 16 nations of the Economic Community of West African States have also prohibited both the import and export of uniodized salt.

After taking such a toll on the mental and physical health of so many and for so long, the iodine problem is therefore now being forced to give ground. WHO and UNICEF have reasonable confidence that, in three or four years from now, the overall goal will be achieved: no more infants will be born as cretins as a result of iodine deficiency; no more parents will suffer the long-drawn-out agony of discovering that their children are severely and permanently retarded; no more sons and daughters will be mentally and physically impaired by this age-old disorder.

Protein-energy nutrition

The world has a strong image of malnutrition. It is the image of a child with eyes too large for a face that is old before its time, a child whose grey and dehydrated skin is drawn taut over a fragile ribcage, a child almost too weak to lift the empty bowl to be filled with food donated from overseas. Staring out from news report or fund-raising advertisement, this is the image that burns itself on our collective conscience like a brand of civilization's failure.

Such malnutrition is real: real in Somalia, real in Rwanda, real in Liberia. But it is unusual and extreme, affecting less than 1% of the developing world's children and almost always as a result of some quite exceptional circumstance - war, or famine, or both.

But there is another malnutrition which is not visible, either to parents or health workers or to a worldwide public. It is the malnutrition of the 1-year-old child who weighs only 6 kilos, of the child who looks to be 7 years old but turns out to be 10 or 11, of the child who is sitting in the shade, dull-eyed, without even the energy to ward off the flies, of the child who rarely joins in the games and adventures of others, of the child whose eyes are glazed over behind a school desk and who does not understand or remember what he or she is being taught. For poor nutrition in the early years of life does not only mean low walls of resistance to disease, or bones that fail to lengthen as they should, or muscles that fail to grow strong, or eyesight that is not as sharp or hearing not as keen. It also means disruption in the miraculous process by which neurons migrate to the right location in the brain and begin to form the billions of subtle synapses that make lifelong learning possible.

This is the protein-energy malnutrition (PEM) that, in some degree, affects vastly greater numbers - over one third of all the children under five in the developing world. It is not caused by the lack of any one particular nutrient, but by the complex interaction of poor diet and frequent illness. And it strikes at the foundations of development in both people and nations. As the World Health Organization has said: *"The nutritional well-being of people is a pre condition for the development of societies ... Governments will be unsuccessful in their efforts to accelerate economic development in any significant long-term sense until optimal child growth and development are ensured for the majority."*[14]

PROMISE: The World Summit for Children acknowledged that today's knowledge could drastically reduce PEM, even at relatively low levels of economic development.[15] Studies supported by UNICEF in recent years have identified the key factors in PEM reduction and shown that it can be achieved at low cost on a large scale. The goal of halving the 1990 rate of child malnutrition by the year 2000 was therefore adopted - and subsequently endorsed by the 1992 International Conference on Nutrition. In order to reach that goal, it was agreed that a reduction of at least 20% would need to be achieved by the end of 1995.

PROGRESS: On the basis of information from 87 developing countries, UNICEF considers that 21 are on track to achieve this mid-decade target (fig. 5). Another 40 could do so with an acceleration of already existing national efforts. Overall, 16 developing nations have now reduced child malnutrition to the point at which fewer than 10% of children are more than two standard deviations below the expected weight-for-age. Although most of these countries are to be found in Latin America and the Caribbean, they also include Egypt and Malaysia. Six more nations - including China and Thailand - have reasonable hopes of falling below that level by the end of 1995. Two countries in sub-Saharan Africa, Tanzania and Zimbabwe, could also see their efforts rewarded by a fall in the malnutrition rate to less than 10% before the middle of this decade.

Progress towards the agreed goal of halving child malnutrition by the year 2000 is therefore being made in over half of the nations of the developing world.

Vitamin A

In 1990, more than half a million mothers first noticed that there was something wrong with their child's eyes. Typically, the first sign of the problem was an inability to see properly in the half-light of dawn or dusk. Soon afterwards, foamy-white specks or patches began to appear in the child's eyes. Wiped away easily at first, they began to recur more frequently. After a few months, the child, obviously weak, fell victim to an attack of diarrhoea or measles from which he or she never seemed to properly recover. Later still, the child began avoiding the light altogether, hardly ever venturing out of doors, and keeping his or her eyes tightly shut for long periods. Finally, the cornea of the eye began to dissolve, and, after three or four more hours, it was gone. Within a year, half of those 500,000 children had died from common diseases which they were clearly too weak to resist. Those who survived will not see again.

Fig. 5 Meeting the mid-decade goals

Number of developing countries on track to achieve the mid-decade goal of reducing 1990 child malnutrition rates by 20%.

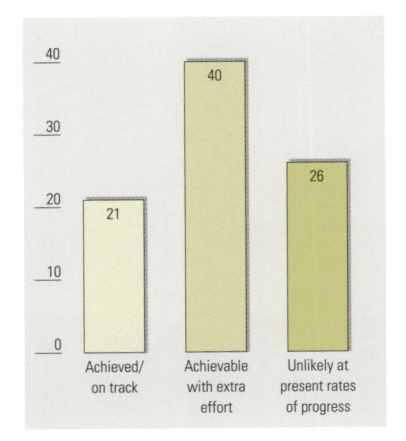

Achieved/on track	Achievable with extra effort	Unlikely at present rates of progress
21	40	26

Source: *Country assessments by UNICEF field staff, for 87 countries, September 1994.*

Fig. 6 Vitamin A deficiency
Estimated impact of vitamin A deficiency on under-fives in the developing world.

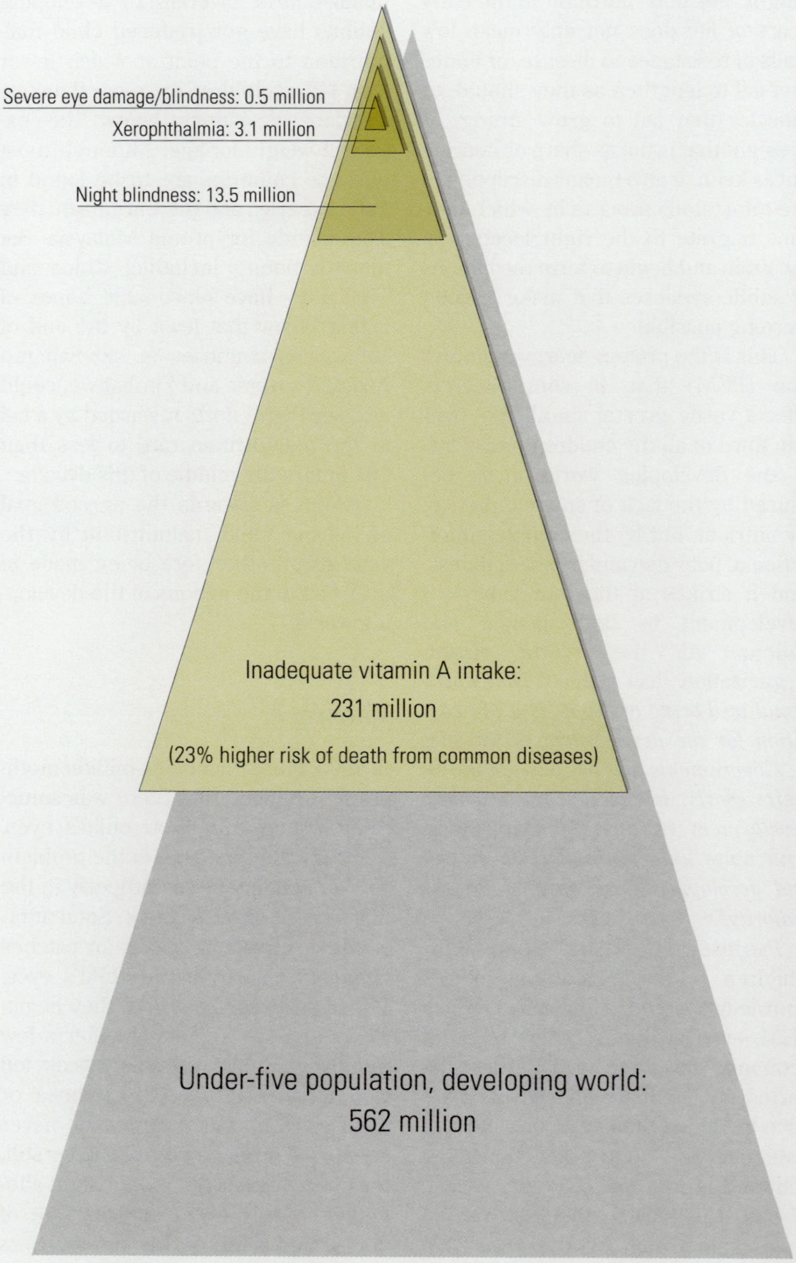

Severe eye damage/blindness: 0.5 million

Xerophthalmia: 3.1 million

Night blindness: 13.5 million

Inadequate vitamin A intake:
231 million

(23% higher risk of death from common diseases)

Under-five population, developing world:
562 million

The clinical signs of xerophthalmia include Bitot's spots on the eye as well as drying, ulcerating and scarring of the cornea. Half of the children who go blind are dead within a few months.

Source: *Adapted from WHO estimates, September 1994.*

The annual tragedy of half a million children losing their sight was only the tip of a very much larger problem.

The cause was vitamin A deficiency. And like iodine deficiency, both problem and solution have been known for decades: daily diets can be changed, usually at little cost, to include small amounts of green leafy vegetables; or 2-cent vitamin A capsules can be given three times a year to children over six months of age; or vitamin A can be added to sugar or cooking oil.

In the mid-1980s, it was discovered that the annual tragedy of those half-million children was the tip of a very much larger problem (fig. 6). Five hundred times that number of children have lowered resistance to disease because of milder forms of the deficiency; and the consequence is death rates that are commonly 20% to 30% higher than in children whose vitamin A intake is adequate.[16]

WHO and UNICEF also brought this issue before the 1990 World Summit for Children - arguing that improving vitamin A intake was another of the obvious, powerful, low-cost strategies with the potential to reduce illness, blindness, and death among the children of the developing world.

PROMISE: As a result, governments of affected countries made a formal commitment to the virtual elimination of vitamin A deficiency by the end of 1995.

PROGRESS: Of the 67 nations concerned, 35 are likely to come close to eliminating the problem by the end of 1995. Approximately two thirds of all the children at risk live in those 35 countries (fig. 7).

Thirty-two other nations have not yet begun to take preventive action on a sufficient scale. But this picture too is changing rapidly: in 1994, Mexico has administered vitamin A supplements to 2.5 million children in 887 high-risk municipalities; Guatemala has already fortified most sugar with vitamin A; Viet Nam has launched a national vitamin A day with the aim of reaching 10 million children.

By mid-decade, these achievements will mean that hundreds of thousands of child deaths from diarrhoea and measles will be prevented each year. These two diseases currently account for nearly half of all the child deaths in the world - and are rendered more deadly by vitamin A deficiency. In addition, at least 200,000 children a year will have their eyesight saved.

Iron

In 1990, four out of ten women in the developing world were suffering from a specific condition causing exhaustion and general poor health. Among pregnant women, more than half were affected - struggling through the difficult months before the birth with hardly enough energy to get through the long daily workload and with little awareness that they faced increased risk of death in childbirth, or that their babies were also at higher risk of low birth weight and impaired development.[17]

The cause was iron deficiency anaemia.

Supplementing iron is relatively simple and inexpensive. Ferrous sulphate tablets must be taken daily, but their cost is less than one fifth of 1 cent each. In the near future, the task should become even more achievable with the discovery that a once-a-week tablet is almost as effective.

PROMISE: At the 1990 World Summit for Children, governments made a commitment to reduce iron deficiency anaemia in women by at least one third of its 1990 level before the end of this century.

PROGRESS: Very few countries have so far taken national-scale action to eliminate iron deficiency anaemia (fig. 8).

India is a major and hopeful exception. Latest reports (1994) indicate that over 70% of women are now being reached with at least three months' worth of ferrous sulphate tablets during pregnancy, and the goal of a one-third reduction in anaemia by the year 2000 is certainly feasible in the country which is home to approximately half of the estimated 466 million women in the world who suffer from iron deficiency anaemia.

Fig. 7 Meeting the mid-decade goals
Number of developing countries on track to achieve the mid-decade goal of eliminating vitamin A deficiency in affected countries.

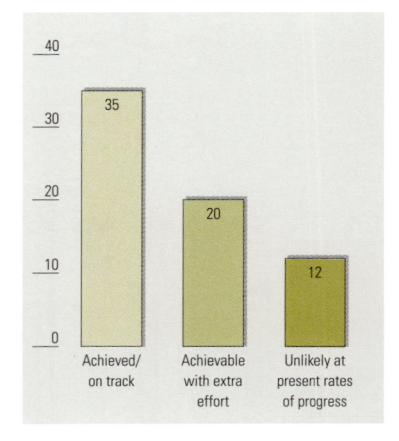

Source: *Country assessments by UNICEF field staff, for 67 countries, September 1994.*

Fig. 8 Anaemia in pregnancy

Percentage of all women and of pregnant women suffering from iron deficiency anaemia.

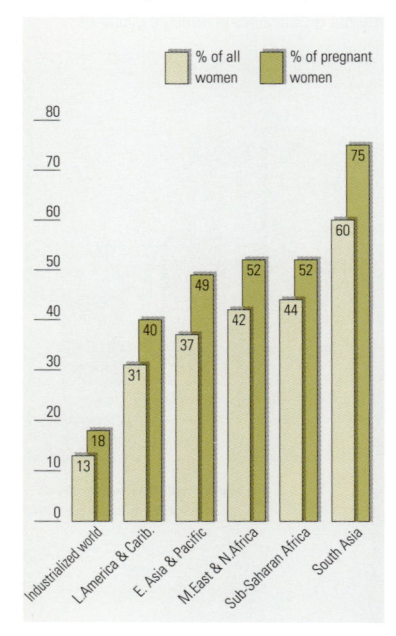

Region	% of all women	% of pregnant women
Industrialized world	13	18
L.America & Carib.	31	40
E. Asia & Pacific	37	49
M.East & N.Africa	42	52
Sub-Saharan Africa	44	52
South Asia	60	75

Source: *Adapted from WHO, The prevalence of anaemia in women: a tabulation of available information, 1992.*

No mid-decade target was established for progress against anaemia; but the goal of virtual elimination before the end of this decade is unlikely to be met without a significant acceleration of effort over the next six years.

Baby-friendly

In 1990, more than 1 million infants died who would not have died if they had been exclusively breastfed for the first six months of their lives.[18] Malnourished and weakened, most of those infants' deaths were marked by the last painful gasps of an acute respiratory infection, or by the sudden and dreadful draining away of life by diarrhoeal disease.

Most of those infants died because they had been fed with breastmilk substitutes. Their parents, often poor and illiterate and living in unhygienic conditions, may have decided to use commercial formula for many reasons, including the need for the mother to work outside the home and leave the baby to be fed by someone else. Many were also persuaded by advertisements, and by the misguided example and advice of hospitals and maternity units.

Commercial infant formulas are an expensive and inferior substitute for breastmilk. They are frequently over-diluted in order to save money, and mixed with unsafe water before being fed to the child from an unsterilized bottle capped with an unclean teat. Exclusive breastfeeding, by contrast, provides complete, hygienic, inexpensive nutrition. It also protects against common diseases and delays the return of ovulation - thereby helping to prevent a new pregnancy following too soon after the last.[19]

One million deaths a year is the measure of these differences.

PROMISE: After two decades of evidence in support of the conclusions outlined above, governments represented at the World Summit for Children made a new commitment to the promotion of breastfeeding.

To make this aim specific and measurable, it was later agreed that the distribution of free and low-cost breastmilk substitutes to hospitals and to maternity wards would be ended in all countries by mid-decade. It was also decided that an attempt would be made to encourage all hospitals and maternity units to adopt the 'ten steps to successful breastfeeding' drawn up in 1989 by an expert group sponsored by WHO and UNICEF under the chairmanship of the then Nigerian Health Minister, Dr. Ransome Kuti.[20]

PROGRESS: The practical results to date are moderately encouraging.

Of the 72 developing countries that previously allowed free or subsidized infant formulas to be distributed in hospitals and maternity clinics, all but one, Kuwait, have banned the practice (as of September 1994).

In 57 out of 102 developing countries, the action taken to date makes it likely that almost all major hospitals (defined as teaching hospitals, provincial hospitals, and other hospitals with more than 1,000 births per year) will have agreed to follow the ten steps to successful breastfeeding by the middle of this decade. In the western hemisphere, the only nations unlikely to achieve the goal are Canada, Haiti, and the United States. In Africa, most of the exceptions are countries affected by war or its aftermath.

In total, almost 1,000 hospitals worldwide are now displaying the 'baby-friendly' plaque which means that they are following the ten steps and do not accept free or low-cost supplies of breastmilk substitutes. In the developing world, over 14,000 hospitals and maternity units are in the process of changing standard procedures to encourage and give practical support to breastfeeding. In the industrialized world, 19 nations have so far set up national authorities to supervise and promote this initiative; in Sweden, 41 out of 61 maternity units were designated 'baby-friendly' by mid-1994.[21]

In the last three years, 30 more countries have taken action on the WHO International Code of Marketing of Breastmilk Substitutes.[22]

Immunization

At the end of the 1970s, fewer than 10% of the world's children were being immunized. Measles, whooping cough, tetanus, and diphtheria were claiming the lives of over 13,000 children every day of every year. Many millions more were being left deaf or blind or crippled by polio and measles, and the nutritional health of even larger numbers was being undermined by preventable diseases that depress the appetite, burn energy in fevers, inhibit the absorption of food, and drain away nutrients in diarrhoea and vomiting.

Against this background, the World Health Assembly set the goal of immunizing 80% of the world's children by the end of 1990.

For a decade, WHO, UNICEF, and many other organizations have worked with governments towards that goal in virtually every village and neighbourhood of Africa, Asia, and Latin America. Its attainment, in the great majority of countries, has meant the prevention of approximately 3 million child deaths a year and the annual prevention of approximately 400,000 cases of polio. "*This extraordinary planetary achievement*," says the WHO Global Advisory Group on immunization, "*is largely unrecognized by the general public.*" [23]

PROMISE: At the World Summit for Children in 1990, the chief concern was that this extraordinary effort, the largest international collaborative effort in peacetime history, might not be sustained. Governments therefore set the goal of maintaining the 80% immunization level (and its achievement by those countries that had not yet done so) in the early years of the 1990s, followed by a raising of immunization levels to 90% or more by the year 2000.

PROGRESS: Immunization figures for 1993 have just become available (mid-1994). By and large they show that the widely feared decline in immunization levels has not occurred (fig. 9). Of the 66 developing nations that achieved the 80% immunization target by the end of 1990, coverage has since increased in 30%, remained stable in 50%, and declined in 20%.[24]

Although forward progress always appears more dramatic, the sustaining of 1990 immunization levels is one of the greatest achievements of the 1990s to date. Immunization levels are in no way cumulative: every year, a new cohort of approximately 140 million newborns must be reached with the right vaccine at the right temperature at the right time on four or five separate occasions during the child's first year of life.

The overall position in 1994 (data for 1993) is set out in figs. 9 and 10. The latest information on the individual target diseases is summarized below.

Polio

Most of the tens of millions of children who were infected by the polio virus in 1990 recovered without ever knowing that they had been attacked. The disease passed without symptom. In some cases, there was a slight fever and some muscle pain which was quickly forgotten. In a small percentage of cases, but a very large absolute number, the fever remained high and the pain became muscle weakness, usually in the larger muscles of the leg. In these cases, the virus was replicating itself and entering the junctions of the motor neurons which control the movements of the muscle.

Some of those children recovered all or most of the lost muscle control over the following three months. But for approximately 200,000 of those children, the virus destroyed 50% or 60% of the neurons serving the muscle, meaning that it could no longer function normally. Permanent paralysis was the result.

For a few of those children, the part of the body that no longer functioned was not the leg but the respiratory system.

PROMISE: The World Summit for Children made a commitment to the eradication of polio by the end of the 1990s. Most of the countries in the

Fig. 9 Immunization coverage

Percentage of the developing world's under-ones protected against five of the major vaccine-preventable diseases.

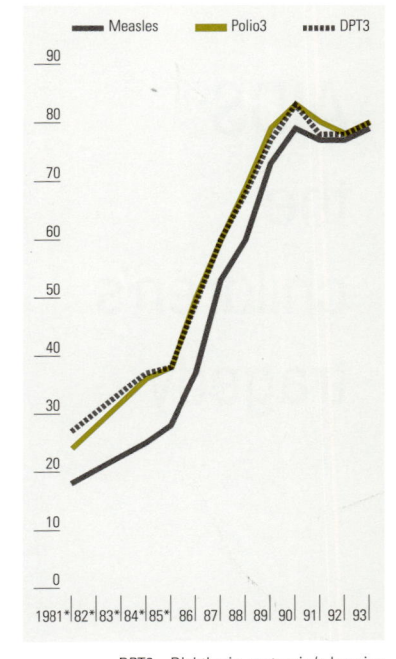

DPT3 = Diphtheria, pertussis (whooping cough), and tetanus vaccine (3 doses).
*Excluding China.
Source: *WHO and UNICEF, September 1994.*

Fig. 10 Meeting the mid-decade goals

Number of developing countries on track to achieve the mid-decade goal of reaching or maintaining an 80% immunization (as measured by the % of under-ones fully immunized).

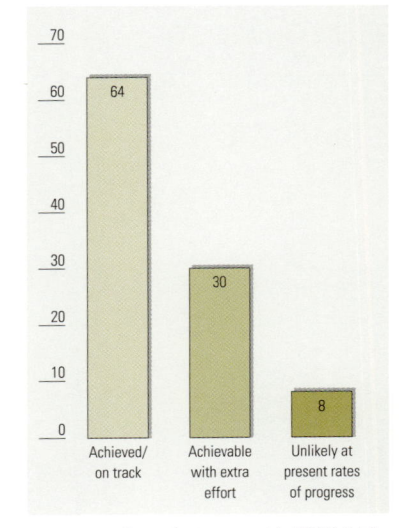

- Achieved/on track: 64
- Achievable with extra effort: 30
- Unlikely at present rates of progress: 8

Source: *Country assessments by UNICEF field staff, for 102 countries, September 1994.*

Panel 5

AIDS: the children's tragedy

"A decade ago, women and children seemed to be on the periphery of the AIDS epidemic. Today, women and children are at the centre of our concern."
WHO Global Programme on AIDS, September 1993.

Worldwide, as many women as men are contracting the AIDS virus. In Africa, women now account for 55% of all new cases of HIV.

As the AIDS epidemic grows, it is becoming clear that women are more vulnerable than men. The reasons are both biological and social. Biologically, women are at more risk because a larger mucosal surface is exposed during sexual intercourse and because semen carries a greater concentration of the virus than vaginal fluid. Socially, they are more vulnerable because they tend to marry or have sex with older men who have had more sexual partners - and because they may have little or no choice about whether and with whom they have sex. Often, women are not in a position either to say no or to influence their partner's sexual behaviour (including whether or not condoms are used).

In some areas of Africa, 25% to 30% of pregnant women attending antenatal clinics are HIV-positive. One in three of their babies will be born with the virus. All will develop AIDS and most will die before the age of five. So far, approximately 1 million children have been infected and half a million have already died - almost all of them in Africa.

HIV is also known to have been transmitted by breastmilk in some instances. But breastfeeding is still recommended in areas where the risk from malnutrition and disease is paramount.

Two thirds of all new cases of HIV are now occurring in Africa, where 9 million children will be orphaned in the 1990s and where recent gains in child survival are being reversed. In Zimbabwe, for example, AIDS has already become the biggest single killer of the nation's under-fives.

But the situation in some countries in Asia is giving almost as much cause for concern. Thailand reports that 1 adult in 50 is infected with HIV, and a study by Mahidol University suggests that the country's under-five mortality rate will rise by 10% before the end of the century.

With no AIDS vaccine in sight, only behavioural change offers hope of altering the course of an epidemic that could see 26 million people infected and an annual death toll of almost 2 million by the year 2000. Sex education for young people (60% of new HIV infections occur in the 15-to-24 age group) is essential. And recent studies have strengthened this case by showing that sex education is not associated with either more or earlier sexual activity.

Even more fundamentally, the growing AIDS threat to women and children will not diminish until women have more power to say no to sex, to choose their own partners, and to influence sexual behaviour.

Resources are also required. Yet of the estimated $2 billion spent annually on AIDS prevention, only about 10% is spent in the developing world, where 85% of infections are occurring. □

western hemisphere, in East Asia, and in the Middle East and North Africa accepted that this goal could be achieved by the end of 1995.

Progress: 43 out of 55 developing nations that have adopted the 1995 target are on track to achieve that goal.

As of August 1994, all of the western hemisphere has been free of polio for at least three years.[25] In achieving this target - under the leadership of the Pan American Health Organization and with strong support from UNICEF, the Canadian International Development Agency, the United States Agency for International Development and Rotary International - several countries have pioneered the strategy of national immunization days to supplement routine immunization programmes. Other nations are now adopting the same approach. China has held national immunization days in 25 provinces and succeeded in reducing the reported number of polio cases from 5,000 in 1990 to 538 in 1993. The Philippines and Viet Nam held immunization days in 1993 and 1994. Iran, Pakistan, and Syria have done the same in 1994. India and Bangladesh will follow in 1995. India, which is phasing in the goal state by state, aims to have eradicated polio from 11 states, with a combined population of 250 million, by the end of 1994.

Worldwide, these achievements are reflected in a steep fall in polio cases. According to WHO estimates,[26] there were almost 400,000 new victims of polio in 1983; by 1994 that total had fallen to just over 100,000 (fig. 11).

If this effort can be sustained, most of the nations of Latin America, East Asia, and North Africa and the Middle East will achieve the goal of polio eradication by the end of 1995. With some increase in outside help, most of the nations of South Asia and sub-Saharan Africa will do so by the year 2000.

By that time, it is likely that there will be at least 5 million children below the age of 10 who will be growing up normally but who would have been paralysed for life by polio were it not for the effort to reach this goal.

Measles

In the mid-1980s, measles was accepted as a normal part of childhood across much of the developing world. Most children recovered within a few days. Many suffered a drop in weight and a loss of vitamin A, making them vulnerable to the cycle of frequent illness and poor growth. Some were left with severe conjunctivitis. Others developed otitis media and are now deaf. But in about 3 million cases a year, the reddish-purple rash of measles grew more severe and the skin began to scale. In some cases, life was drained away in severe diarrhoea and dehydration. In others, the end came with convulsions or bronchial pneumonia. In others, the child's pulse rate continued to rise as high as 180 before the heart gave way. In all 3 million cases, death was the result of one of the most common and easily prevented of childhood's diseases.

Promise: The 1990 Summit called for a 95% reduction in measles deaths (compared with pre-immunization levels).

Progress: WHO and UNICEF believe that a majority of developing nations are likely to achieve the goal of a 95% reduction by the end of 1995.

According to assessments made in mid-1994 by UNICEF representatives in 102 developing countries, the goal is likely to be achieved in over 54 countries, and could be achieved in 38 more with an acceleration of existing efforts. Of the 10 nations unlikely to meet the goal, 7 are in sub-Saharan Africa.

If the 1995 goal is achieved, this will bring the annual number of child deaths from measles down to fewer than half a million, as opposed to more than 1 million in 1990, 3 million in the mid-1980s, and 7 to 8 million before measles vaccination began (fig. 12).

Although the measles immunization level for the developing world as a whole remains high at 79%, this average masks differences between countries that are maintaining or increasing coverage and those that are permitting coverage to slip. In total, 27 countries have let immunization levels fall by

Fig. 11 Warding off polio

Changes in the estimated numbers of polio cases in the developing world (in thousands) compared with changes in polio immunization of under-ones.

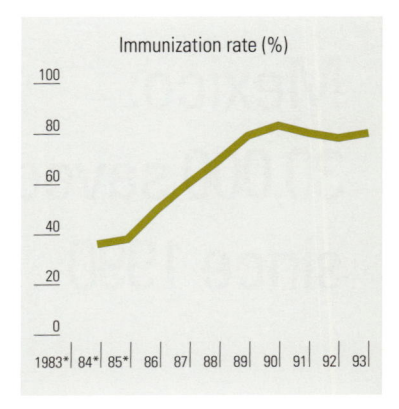

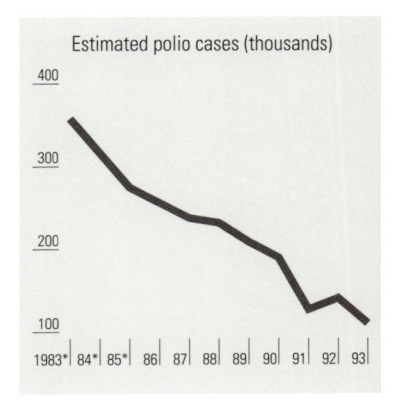

The total number of under-fives in the developing world has increased by approximately 20% since 1983.

*Excluding China.

Source: *WHO and UNICEF, September 1994.*

Panel 6

Mexico: 30,000 saved since 1990

In three years, Mexico has halved child deaths from diarrhoeal disease. An independent evaluation completed in September 1994 shows a 56% fall in diarrhoea deaths among under-five deaths (1990 to 1993).* This means that approximately 30,000 young lives have been saved so far as a result of Mexico's attempts to achieve the 1995 goal of 80% ORT use set by the 1990 World Summit for Children.

In the four years following the Summit, President Carlos Salinas de Gortari gave particular support to the goal of educating all Mexican families in the use of oral rehydration therapy (ORT), the simple and low-cost technique that can prevent most deaths from diarrhoeal disease.

By the end of 1993, over 5 million mothers in Mexico had been trained in ORT. In the worst affected areas, the Ministry of Health has trained approximately 1 million women as health representatives - able to teach others how to prevent and treat the dehydration which turns ordinary diarrhoea into a killer disease.

The training is kept as simple as possible, and is based on three lessons which are known in Spanish as the 'ABC' formula - *alimentación* (continued feeding), *bebidas* (frequent drinks), and *consulta oportuna* (medical help when necessary).

National oral rehydration days and child health weeks have helped to spread these basic messages to virtually every village and urban neighbourhood in Mexico. In 1993 alone, ORT 'advertisements' appeared 120,000 times on national television and more than 2.3 million times on radio. In the same year, almost 8 million posters, pamphlets, and leaflets carried the ORT message under the title 'The best solution'.

To meet the increased demand generated by these campaigns, Mexico's annual production of oral rehydration salts has increased from 9 million packets in 1989 to 83 million in 1993.

To back up the mass education campaigns, health workers and doctors in both government service and private practice have been trained in the correct case management of diarrhoeal disease. Investment in clean water and safe sanitation has been increased, and a system has been set up to monitor diarrhoeal infections more closely.

As a result of all of these efforts, the estimated incidence of diarrhoeal disease in young children has declined from 3.5 to 2.2 episodes per child per year. In the cases that still occur, the use of ORT has increased from 66% to over 80% (and of the specially formulated oral rehydration salts from 22% to 42%).

So far, health authorities from 45 developing countries have visited Mexico to study a campaign which is defeating the number one killer of the nation's children and taking Mexico a long way towards the overall year 2000 target of a one-third reduction in under-five deaths. □

* The evaluation was undertaken by a team of experts from WHO, the Pan American Health Organization, the United States Agency for International Development, the US Centers for Disease Control, Harvard University, and UNICEF.

5 percentage points or more since 1990 and are in danger of allowing the achievement of the measles goal to slip from their grasp.

Neonatal tetanus

In 1990, neonatal tetanus was held to be responsible for over 700,000 infant deaths each year.* Most of its victims were newborn babies, and very few of them were ever seen by a health worker. In many cases, neither death nor birth was officially registered.

Tetanus is therefore the most hidden of diseases, and the one that impinges least on the lives of the more fortunate. But it is not hidden from the parents of those half-million infants upon whom tetanus lays its cold grip.

Cruelly, the first symptom is often taken to be the baby's first smile. But someone in the family soon notices that the smile is fixed and strangely contorted. All that day the tiny jaw muscles stiffen further until the baby cannot open its mouth wide enough even to breastfeed. Hungry and attempting to cry, the infant's temperature rises. The next day the infant is shuddering with muscle spasms, the ghastly smile still in place as the toxin slowly seeps through the nervous system into the spinal cord and the cranial nerves. Racked by cramp-like pains, the spasms increase, the baby's limbs bent but stiff, tiny fists clenched, toes flexing and unflexing, until, towards the end of the second day, the spasms have become uncontrollable and congestion begins to build in liver, lungs, and brain. Out of sight of the world, a brief life comes to an end, writhing in the pitiless arms of a disease which the world has long known how to prevent.

PROMISE: The World Summit for Children adopted the goal of virtually eliminating neonatal tetanus (NT) by the end of 1995.

PROGRESS: In mid-1994, WHO reported: *"The 1995 goal of neonatal tetanus elimination has been achieved in many countries and districts and will be achieved by more, but the target will not be achieved everywhere unless routine coverage is sustained and immunization activities in all high-risk districts are accelerated."* [27]

Similarly, a mid-1994 review by UNICEF suggests that 50 out of 100 developing countries are on target to achieve the NT goal by the end of 1995 (fig. 13). Possibly as many as 32 more countries could do so with a major renewal of effort over the next 12 months. Of the 18 in which the goal is unlikely to be met, 12 are in sub-Saharan Africa.

Diarrhoea and pneumonia

The 1990 Summit also announced targets for the attack on the two most common causes of illness and death among the children of the developing world - pneumonia and diarrhoea. Each of these claims approximately 3 million young lives a year. Together, they account for nearly half of all deaths under the age of five. Both are susceptible to relatively simple and inexpensive solutions. Most deaths from pneumonia could be prevented by the early prescription of low-cost antibiotics. Most deaths from diarrhoeal disease could be prevented by almost cost-free oral rehydration therapy (ORT) and continued feeding.

PROMISE: Confronted with these facts, political leaders at the 1990 Summit adopted the goals of a one-third reduction in child deaths from acute respiratory infections and a halving of child deaths from diarrhoeal disease by the year 2000.

To reach the goal of reducing deaths from diarrhoeal dehydration, it was further agreed that all families would be informed about ORT, and that 80% should be empowered to use the technique by the end of 1995.

PROGRESS: The most recent figures (1993) on progress towards this goal suggest that the ORT use rate was at that time approximately 44% for the developing world as a whole. Latin America led with 64%, followed by the Middle East and North Africa at 55%. Sub-Saharan Africa was nearing 50%. South Asia stood at approximately 40%,

Fig. 12 Protection against measles

Changes in under-five deaths from measles in the developing world (in millions) compared with changes in measles immunization of under-ones.

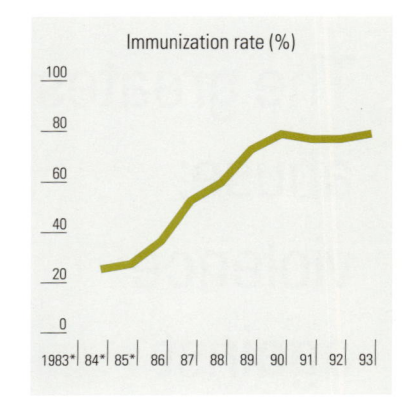

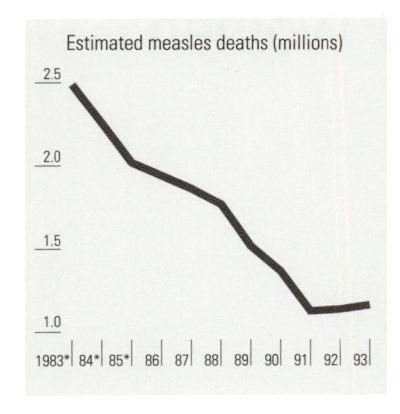

The total number of under-fives in the developing world has increased by approximately 20% since 1983.

*Excluding China.

Source: *WHO and UNICEF, September 1994.*

* Estimates of neonatal tetanus deaths have recently been increased as a result of evidence that tetanus remains a major problem in China, where it claims an estimated 100,000 infant lives each year.

Panel 7

The greatest abuse: violence against women

The death of half a million women a year in pregnancy and childbirth is described in this report as one of the least-protested scandals of the late 20th century. But it is rivalled by another of the great hidden issues - the violence inflicted on women by their male partners.

Surveys in recent years indicate that about a quarter of the world's women are violently abused in their own homes. Community-based surveys have yielded higher figures - up to 50% in Thailand, 60% in Papua New Guinea and the Republic of Korea, and 80% in Pakistan and Chile. In the United States, domestic violence is the biggest single cause of injury to women, accounting for more hospital admissions than rapes, muggings, and road accidents combined.

Such figures suggest that assaults on women by their husbands or male partners are the world's most common form of violence.

The problem is as difficult to solve as it is to measure - and for the same reason. Almost always, the violence occurs within the privacy of the home - into which friends, relations, neighbours, and authorities are reluctant to intrude. The victims themselves voice fewer complaints, and have less recourse to the law, than other victims of violence.

Many of the victims come to accept beatings as an inevitable accompaniment of a woman's inferior status in home and society. Conditioned from birth to esteem themselves only in terms of their ability to serve and satisfy others, many women respond to violence by looking first to their own failings, blaming themselves, justifying their attackers, and hiding the marks of their shame, the tears and the bruises, from the outside world. Often, self-esteem will sink so low that the victim will isolate herself from friends and family - and from the knowledge that she deserves better.

Children also suffer. A mother who is a victim of domestic violence is twice as likely to have a miscarriage and four times more likely to have a low-birth-weight baby. Her children are also more likely to be malnourished, to drop out of school, and to become violent in their turn. More widely, violence against women is also a tragedy for development efforts. As a recent UNICEF publication puts it, the enormous contribution that a woman makes to family, community, and national life depends upon "*her knowledge and strength, her morale and personal relationships, the support of her family and community, her participation in the affairs of the wider world, and her sense of command over the forces shaping her life.*" Domestic violence devastates all of these.

In more and more countries, attempts are being made to bring this problem into the open, to help the victims, and to expose the causes. In Latin America alone, there are over 400 non-governmental organizations specifically concerned with violence against women.

Two recent publications, published by the UN Development Fund for Women and the World Bank, have attempted to assess the scale and impact of this problem.* One disturbing feature of such research is the possibility of a link between domestic violence and progress towards equality for women (as measured, for example, by the closing of the literacy gap between males and females). The suspicion is that the risk of violence rises when male partners feel that their traditional position of superiority and control is being threatened. □

---

* Roxanna Carrillo, *Battered dreams: violence against women as an obstacle to development*, United Nations Development Fund for Women (UNIFEM), New York, 1992; and Lori Heise with Jacqueline Pitanguy and Adrienne Germain, *Violence against women: the hidden health burden*, discussion paper, World Bank, Population, Health, and Nutrition Department, Washington, D.C., 1994.

and East Asia had reached 36% (63% if China is excluded). These figures compare with use rates of almost zero in the early 1980s (fig. 14).

Progress to date means that more than 1 million deaths a year are being prevented.

Estimates from UNICEF offices in 1994 suggest that the situation is still changing quickly, and that 44 developing nations are on track to achieve the 80% target by the end of 1995 (fig. 15). That goal has already been reached in 17 countries: Argentina, Bhutan, Cameroon, Chile, Cuba, the Democratic People's Republic of Korea, Guinea, Iran, Libya, Mexico (panel 6), Saudi Arabia, Syria, the United Arab Emirates, Uruguay, Venezuela, Zambia, and Zimbabwe. Seven countries - Indonesia, Kenya, Lesotho, Namibia, Sri Lanka, Tanzania, and Trinidad and Tobago - are all reported to be very close to 80% as at mid-1994.

Even more important, from the point of view of reducing deaths from diarrhoeal disease, most countries are making rapid progress in the use of the specially formulated oral rehydration salts (ORS) that are needed in cases of diarrhoeal disease severe enough for the parents to seek qualified help.[28]

Much less progress can be reported in the struggle against acute respiratory infections. A simple case-management strategy has been developed by WHO to enable health workers to diagnose and treat pneumonia safely and economically using low-cost antibiotics. Wherever this strategy has been implemented, pneumonia deaths have fallen sharply. But few large-scale national efforts have been mounted. And although antibiotics are effective and inexpensive, the problem of getting them to the right children at the right time is proving difficult to overcome - as is the resistance of the medical profession to the idea that community health workers should be authorized to prescribe the necessary antibiotics.

The year 2000 goal of reducing child deaths from pneumonia by one third is therefore unlikely to be met without a significant acceleration of progress in the remaining years of the 1990s.

If no advance is made on the situation as it stood in 1990, then the number of children under five who will die unnecessarily from pneumonia in this last decade of the 20th century will be approximately 30 million - more than the entire child population of the European Community or of the United States and Canada.[29]

Dracunculiasis

In 1990, dracunculiasis or guinea worm disease was bringing months of pain, infected ulcers, fever, and joint deformities to approximately 3 million people in Africa and Asia. It meant temporary disability to many, and permanent disability to some. And it was having a measurable impact on both productivity and educational attainment (in the acute phase of the disease, the pain is too severe for victims to either work or go to school).

PROMISE: The governments of all affected countries agreed to attempt the eradication of dracunculiasis by the end of 1995.

PROGRESS: Victory over dracunculiasis is imminent. Surveillance data from 1993 show a 25% reduction over 1992 in the number of villages where the disease is considered endemic (fig. 16).[30] India, with over 23,000 cases in 1986, had fewer than 800 in 1993. Pakistan saw only 2 cases in just one village in the whole of 1993. Cameroon reported only 72 cases in the whole of 1993. Uganda reduced its number of cases by 60% (from about 126,000 to a reported 43,000) in the first year of its intervention programme, and there is every likelihood that the disease will soon be eliminated nationwide. Ghana has reduced cases by 90% since 1990. Nigeria recorded over 183,000 cases in 1992 and only 76,000 in 1993.

Overall, the figures suggest that the total number of people suffering from guinea worm disease is now under half a million - a reduction of nearly 90%

Fig. 13 Neonatal tetanus

Tetanus immunization of pregnant women in the developing world compared with changes in infant deaths from tetanus (in millions).

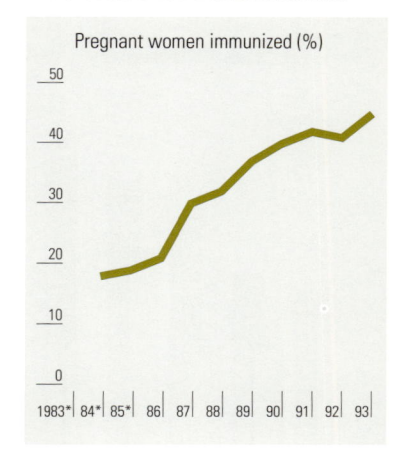

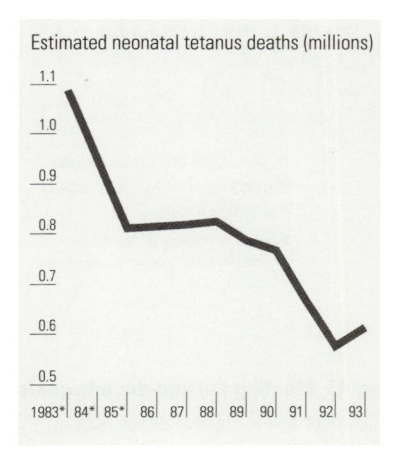

Pregnant women immunized (%)

Estimated neonatal tetanus deaths (millions)

As well as killing over half a million newborns, tetanus causes the deaths of more than 50,000 mothers a year.

The total number of births in the developing world has increased by approximately 20% since 1983.

*Excluding China.

Source: *WHO and UNICEF, September 1994.*

Fig. 14 The rise of ORT

Percentage of diarrhoea bouts in under-fives treated with oral rehydration in the developing world.

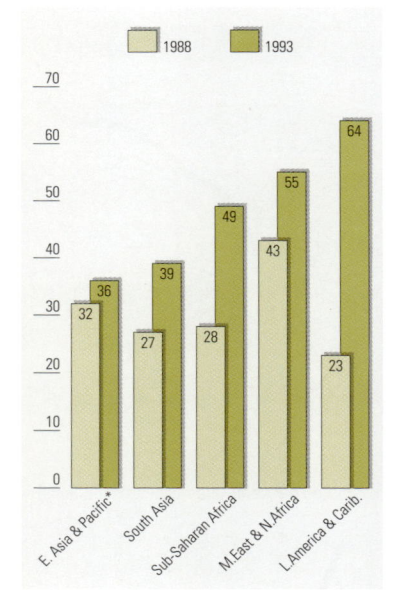

Region	1988	1993
E. Asia & Pacific*	32	36
South Asia	27	39
Sub-Saharan Africa	28	49
M.East & N.Africa	43	55
L.America & Carib.	23	64

*If China (22% ORT use) is excluded, the 1993 figure for East Asia and the Pacific rises to 63%.

Source: *WHO, Programme for Control of Diarrhoeal Diseases, Interim programme reports, relevant years.*

Fig. 15 Meeting the mid-decade goals

Number of developing countries on track to achieve the mid-decade goal of ensuring 80% ORT use for diarrhoeal disease.

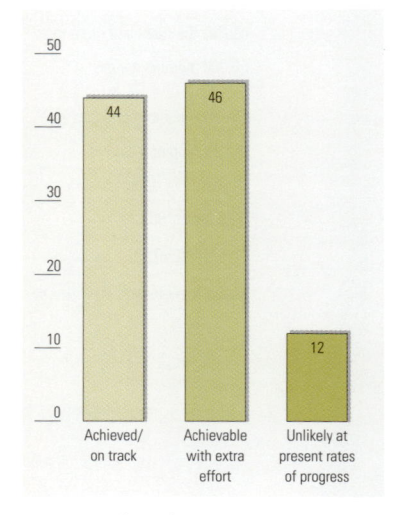

Achieved/on track	44
Achievable with extra effort	46
Unlikely at present rates of progress	12

Source: *Country assessments by UNICEF field staff, for 102 countries, September 1994.*

since the late 1980s. There is every chance that, by the end of 1995, guinea worm disease will be gone from Asia and most of Africa, leaving the problem concentrated in West Africa and in the strife-torn areas in and around southern Sudan.

If achieved, success against guinea worm disease will be a result of a joint effort between governments, UNICEF, WHO, the Carter Center's Global 2000 programme, the WHO Collaborating Center at the US Centers for Disease Control, the World Bank, and other institutions and organizations.

Maternal mortality

In 1990, approximately half a million women died from causes related to pregnancy, abortion, and childbirth. According to the best available estimates, 70,000 of those women died as a result of illegal and unsafe abortion. For every woman who died, several more survived with injuries, diseases, and disabilities which were often painful, embarrassing, and untreated.

PROMISE: The 1990 Summit set the goal of halving, by the year 2000, deaths from causes related to pregnancy, abortion, and childbirth.

PROGRESS: So far, there is little practical progress to report. In part, this may be because most statistics on maternal mortality date from the 1980s. But there is no reason to believe that any significant inroads have been made into this problem in the 1990s, and there is some evidence that maternal mortality has been increasing in sub-Saharan Africa.[31]

In the main, the lack of progress is related to the belief that the problem of maternal mortality can only be reduced by the kind of advanced emergency obstetric care which is only available in major hospitals. This is no longer true. As the Director-General of WHO, Dr. Hiroshi Nakajima, has noted in 1994, *"most of the conditions that result in neonatal death and severe morbidity can be prevented or treated without resorting to sophisticated and expensive technology."*[32] In most countries, the year 2000 goal could still be achieved by a greater awareness of the problem and by relatively low-cost programmes to train and equip existing district hospitals. Most deaths in childbirth occur a long time after a problem has become evident. And there is an urgent need for a much wider and keener awareness - among communities as well as governments, families as well as health services - that all pregnancies involve risk and that immediate transfer to the nearest hospital is essential at the first sign of haemorrhage or abnormal difficulty in labour. As UNICEF has argued before, this is one obvious and practical area where men can begin to assume more responsibility for the health and well-being of their families: wherever possible, all fathers-to-be should make the necessary arrangements, in advance, in case transfer to a hospital becomes necessary during labour.

The September 1994 Cairo International Conference on Population and Development, which gave the issue of women's reproductive health such a central place in its discussions, has done all that a conference can to make the breakthrough on this issue (panel 1). And there is no possible justification for any further delay in tackling the tragedy of maternal mortality. The fact that 1,500 women are being allowed to die each and every day of each and every year from 'maternal causes' is one of the least-protested scandals of the late 20th century. The great majority of those deaths can be prevented by a combination of improved family planning services, a wider awareness of the need for immediate hospitalization if problems arise, and more training of district-level hospital staff to provide emergency obstetric care (including Caesarean section). As the Cairo Conference did so much to make clear, the issue of women's reproductive health is a critical issue both for human rights and social development.

Present levels of maternal mortality are a tragic measure of our failure so far.

Education

Thanks to extraordinary efforts during the 1960s and 1970s, the percentage of children reaching grade 5 (i.e. completing at least four years of primary school) had reached 50% or more in almost all developing countries. But in the 1980s, mounting debts and consequent structural adjustment programmes led many governments to freeze or cut educational spending. As UNESCO has noted,[33] primary schooling often suffered disproportionately, and there was significant slippage in sub-Saharan Africa (fig. 17). Following the 1990 World Conference on Education for All in Jomtien, Thailand, many nations began to give greater priority to universalizing primary education. Also at that time, the World Bank committed itself to a major increase in lending.

PROMISE: The World Summit for Children confirmed the goal of basic education for all children - girls as well as boys - and primary school education for at least 80% by the year 2000.

PROGRESS: In many nations, progress appears to be being resumed. Figures for 1993 suggest that the proportion of the developing world's children now completing at least four years of primary schooling has reached 71% overall.

According to a mid-1994 review by UNICEF, 42 of 95 countries have achieved or are on target to achieve the 1995 goal of a one-third reduction in the gap between 1990 primary school completion rates and the 80% target set for the year 2000 (fig. 18). New commitments to the 80% goal have been made in 1993 and 1994 by the Presidents or Prime Ministers of nine of the most populous nations of the developing world. China, Indonesia and Mexico have already achieved a minimum of four years of schooling for at least 80% of their children. Brazil, Egypt and India could reach the goal if the accelerated efforts now being made in all three countries are continued. Bangladesh, Nigeria, and particularly Pakistan face a massive - but not impossible - task; all three have renewed the effort to expand primary education in the 1990s. Meanwhile, the World Bank has honoured the promise of Jomtien by tripling lending for primary education to nearly $1 billion a year in 1993.[34]

Water and sanitation

The lack of clean water and safe sanitation is one of the greatest of all divides between the absolute poor and the rest of humanity.

In urban slums, in particular, the lack of adequate sanitation devastates the quality of life. Under the heat, flies and smells and disease are dominant and permanent. Frequently, quarrels break out as tensions rise in the long lines for a trickling standpipe that must do for 200 or 300 people. In rural areas, the coming of the dry season is dreaded by millions of women who must then begin walking long distances for unreliable supplies of unsafe water. In the African Sahel, for example, a woman may walk four or five hours a day to fetch one jar, sometimes travelling by night with other women. If she arrives too late, there will be long queues; if she arrives too early, she will probably find that the well has been locked to prevent anyone from taking too much water during the night. After taking a drink from the well and covering the jar with a cloth, she will balance it carefully on the coil of rope on her head and begin the journey home. For several hours more she will walk, swaying gracefully in the picturesque way that all the world has seen in photographs which do not capture the pain in the shoulders and the small of the back. Once home, the liquid may be filtered through a nylon cloth to remove some of the insects and larvae. A small amount will then be used to make millet or sorghum porridge and a sauce. Before the meal, hands will be wiped with minute amounts of water; afterwards the plates will be scrubbed with leaves or ash and then rinsed with more water which is then saved for washing bodies.

PROMISE: The 1990 Summit set the

Fig. 16 Tackling guinea worm
Percentage of villages with endemic dracunculiasis having one or more control interventions at the end of 1993.

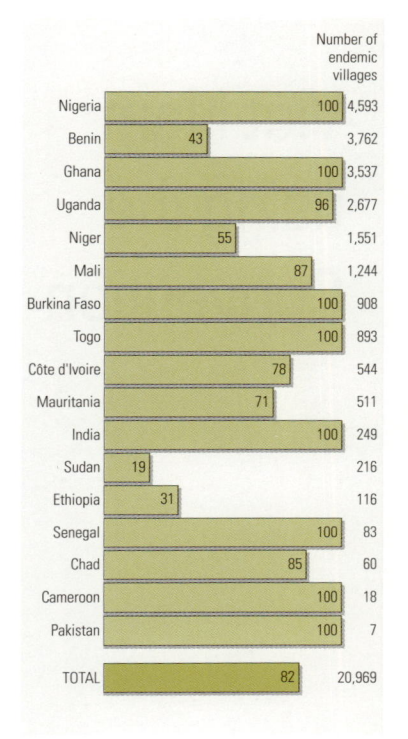

Country	%	Number of endemic villages
Nigeria	100	4,593
Benin	43	3,762
Ghana	100	3,537
Uganda	96	2,677
Niger	55	1,551
Mali	87	1,244
Burkina Faso	100	908
Togo	100	893
Côte d'Ivoire	78	544
Mauritania	71	511
India	100	249
Sudan	19	216
Ethiopia	31	116
Senegal	100	83
Chad	85	60
Cameroon	100	18
Pakistan	100	7
TOTAL	82	20,969

Incidence in Kenya is being assessed.
Figures for Chad, Ethiopia and the Sudan are estimates.

Source: *WHO Collaborating Center for Research, Training, and Eradication of Dracunculiasis at the US Centers for Disease Control,* Guinea worm wrap-up, no. 42, January 1994.

Panel 8

Viet Nam: using the Convention

In less than five years, 167 nations have ratified the Convention on the Rights of the Child - making it the most widely and rapidly ratified convention in history.

But can the Convention help improve children's lives in practice? Viet Nam, the first Asian country to ratify the Convention, is showing that the answer is yes.

The transition from a command to a market economy has produced major economic progress in Viet Nam. It has also produced serious social problems. Levels of child labour, abuse, and delinquency have all risen alarmingly. While statistics are weak, there are now believed to be some 22,000 street children and perhaps 20,000 child prostitutes in Viet Nam.

The Government of Viet Nam expressed its concern, but was poorly equipped to combat these new problems. Legislation concerning children was inadequate and outdated. Police and prison officials lacked training in working with children. Social workers were few and usually unskilled. Non-governmental organizations experienced in child welfare did not exist.

In addition, as the Government itself reported, "*feudal attitudes*" often resulted in discrimination against girls, and in a high priority on obedience combined with a low priority on dialogue with children.

After ratifying the Convention in September 1990, the first major task was the preparation of a report for the Geneva-based Committee on the Rights of the Child (CRC). The Viet Nam Committee for Protection and Care of Children - a governmental body drawing its staff from various ministries and mass organizations - was given responsibility for preparing the first report. UNICEF was requested to assist in meeting the CRC's detailed reporting guidelines, and to help promote public awareness of Viet Nam's obligations under the Convention.

As the drafts became more concrete, the Government gained in confidence, placing increasingly candid emphasis on children in especially difficult circumstances (such as child prostitution), as well as on shortfalls in the overall levels of child health, nutrition, and education.

Reviewing the final text, in early 1993, the CRC congratulated Viet Nam on the report's openness and comprehensive approach, as well as on its willingness to engage in "*constructive and frank dialogue.*"

The CRC also expressed satisfaction with Viet Nam's national plan of action for children 1991-2000, developed following its participation in the 1990 World Summit for Children. Viet Nam is now in the process of developing provincial plans of action in all of its 53 provinces.

Already Viet Nam has taken its first steps to bring national law and policy into harmony with the Convention. Within a two-year period, laws covering the protection, care and education of children, the universalization of primary education, and the protection of public health have all been passed. At the same time, the Government's overall plan - the strategy for socio-economic stabilization and development - calls for a careful watch on child education, culture, and health as the country moves from the current crisis towards more stable development.

The next challenge was the CRC's recommendation for amendments to Viet Nam's penal code on juvenile justice. The Government responded positively, inviting two CRC members to visit Viet Nam as advisers. Swedish Save the Children was requested to provide assistance that would improve laws relating to the imprisonment of delinquent children and the rights of accused children.

The process is still under way. New laws will be formulated, along with plans for training of law enforcement officials and, most importantly, of social workers.

"*Viet Nam has made an extraordinary effort, both to commit itself to reaching the highest international standards, and to begin the hard climb towards those standards,*" says Stephen Woodhouse, the UNICEF Representative in Hanoi. □

goal of access to clean water and safe sanitation for all communities by the year 2000.

PROGRESS: Definitions of 'access' are too varied and statistics too weak to assess how widely that goal is being achieved. Reports from 93 nations suggest that progress commensurate with reaching the goal of clean water for all is being made in approximately 40 countries (fig. 19). For safe sanitation, perhaps only a third of the developing countries are likely to reach the goal on present trends.

This effort is a continuation of the International Drinking Water Supply and Sanitation Decade (1981-1990), which saw the proportion of families with access to safe drinking water rise from 38% to 66% in South-East Asia, from 66% to 80% in Latin America, and from 32% to 42% in Africa.[35] In India, the percentage of rural people with access to safe water has risen from just over 30% in 1980 to about 80% in 1992, and on present trends will reach almost 100% by 1997 or 1998. Similarly, more than a decade of effort against enormous odds has brought Bangladesh to the point where 80% of the rural population now lives within 150 metres of a source of safe drinking water.

By any standards, these are enormous achievements. And they have been brought about despite the fact that only about a fifth of the $10 billion to $12 billion spent on water supply every year is allocated to low-cost water and sanitation schemes serving the poorest communities. With even a partial reordering of such expenditures in favour of the poor, today's knowledge and today's technologies could achieve the goals of clean water and safe sanitation for all in the remaining years of this century.

The Convention

The Convention on the Rights of the Child is widely considered to be the most progressive, detailed, and specific human rights treaty ever adopted by the Member States of the United Nations. By incorporating the right of every child to survive and to develop normally, and to receive at least basic health care and a primary education, the Convention bridges, for the first time, the ideological gap which has always separated economic and social rights from civil and political rights. And it stands as an internationally agreed minimum standard for the treatment of children everywhere.[36]

PROMISE: The governments represented at the World Summit for Children committed themselves to the ratification of the Convention on the Rights of the Child. Subsequently, at the 1993 World Conference on Human Rights in Vienna, it was agreed that universal ratification could and should be achieved by the end of 1995.

PROGRESS: In less than five years, the vast majority of the world's nations - 167 altogether - have ratified the Convention on the Rights of the Child. Nine more have signed the document - indicating an intention to ratify in the near future. Only 14 nations (including Saudi Arabia and the United States) have neither signed nor ratified as of fall 1994.

There is therefore a reasonable chance that the goal will be achieved and that the Convention on the Rights of the Child will become the first human rights treaty in history to be universally ratified.

After ratification, the next step is the preparation of a national report on the measures taken to implement the Convention. These reports, submitted to the Committee on the Rights of the Child, are helping to open up a dialogue on many issues that have previously been either neglected or hidden from the light of discussion. In some cases, the reports have prompted national debate on such issues as street children or child prostitution. In others, countries have been prepared to compare policies and discuss such subjects internationally for the first time. So far, 46 nations have fulfilled the commitment to report in detail on the implementation of the Convention on the Rights of the Child. Panel 8 takes the example of Viet Nam to show this process at work.

Fig. 17 Primary school enrolment
Percentage of 6-11-year-olds enrolled in school.

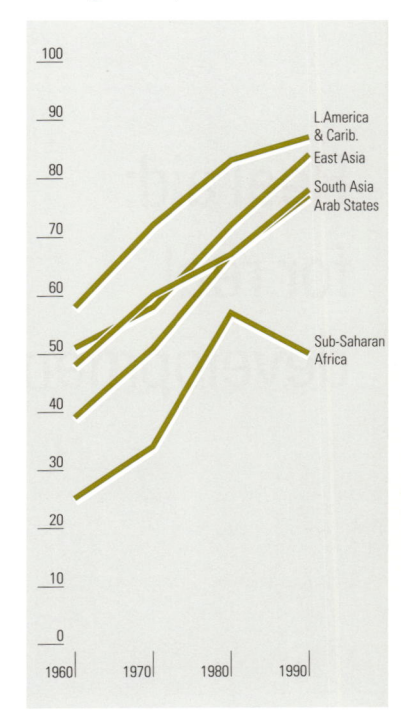

Source: UNESCO, Trends and projections of enrolment by level of education, by age and by sex, 1960-2025, 1993. Based on UNESCO regions.

Fig. 18 Meeting the mid-decade goals
Number of developing countries on track to achieve the mid-decade goal of reducing the primary education shortfall by one third.

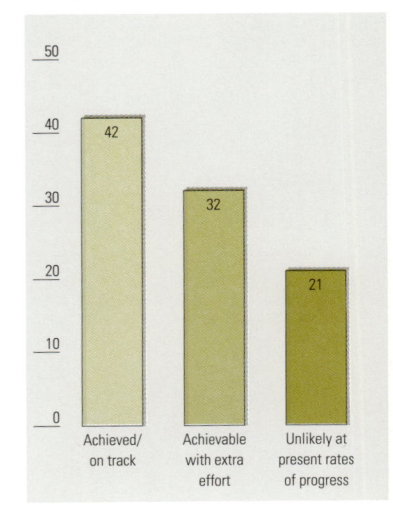

Source: Country assessments by UNICEF field staff, for 95 countries, September 1994.

Panel 9

Real aid: for real development

One of the ways in which people and organizations in the industrialized nations can become involved in implementing today's development consensus is through supporting increases in, and a redirecting of, government aid programmes. Six years ago, the 1989 *State of the World's Children* report made the case for that support:

Public idealism is not dead. Many would march in the cause of abolishing from our planet the worst aspects of absolute poverty - mass malnutrition, preventable illness, and illiteracy. But this idealistic conception of aid is in an advanced state of corrosion. (*Six years on, 25% of the assistance given goes to the 40 least developed countries; less than 15% goes to the agricultural sector; less than 6% goes to primary health care and family planning combined; and only 2% goes to the primary schools that cater for the majority.*)

The one criterion which matters most to the majority of people in both rich and poor worlds is the question of whether aid is helping to overcome the worst aspects of absolute poverty. Is priority given where need is greatest - to the poorest countries and the poorest within countries? Is a significant proportion of aid being used to assist projects in which the poor themselves participate? Is aid being used to improve the lives and lighten the workloads of women? Is aid contributing to environmental degradation or to sustainable development? Is aid helping to finance the recurrent costs and smaller budget items, the textbooks and essential drugs, in order to make efficient use of existing facilities? Is aid being spent on low-cost, high-impact, mass-application strategies which are of primary relevance to meeting the needs and increasing the productivity of the poor?

In sum, aid for development should be real aid for real development.

The ultimate aim and measure of real development is the enhancement of the capacities of the poorest, their health and nutrition, their education and skills, their abilities to meet their own needs, control their own lives, and earn a fair reward for their labours.

And the time has come when not only aid but also debt reduction and trade agreements should form part of a real development pact by which participating industrialized nations would make a commitment to increase resources and participating developing nations would make a corresponding commitment to a pattern of real development that unequivocally puts the poor first.

This is the kind of development which the majority of people in the poor world seek; and this is the kind of development which the majority of people in the industrialized world would support.*

Finally, the under-fives should occupy a special place in real development. For if children are deprived of the chance to grow to their full physical and mental potential, of the opportunity to go to school and learn new skills, and of the chance of a childhood in which love and security predominate over fear and instability, then future progress is constantly being undermined by present poverty. The growing minds and bodies of children must therefore be given priority protection. There could be no greater humanitarian cause; there could be no more productive investment; and there could be no greater priority for real development. □

* Recent surveys of public opinion in the 1990s have confirmed that most people in the industrialized nations favour aid given to help the poor and support health and education, rather than aid given for foreign policy reasons or in support of donor exports.

No one would or should claim that the Convention on the Rights of the Child has yet transformed the reality of child rights abuse. Children continue to go hungry, to succumb to preventable disease, to be denied even an elementary education. They continue to be abused in the home, in the workplace, and in wars. They continue to be exploited, prostituted, raped, and sold, in many of the countries where the Convention has been solemnly signed.

But a universally accepted code for the treatment of children is a major step forward. It provides an unchallengeable platform for advocacy and action on behalf of children in all countries and in all circumstances, and it prepares the way for the next and obviously more difficult stage - the stage of moving from universal acceptance to universal observance.

Finally, the unusual nature of this Convention should not be forgotten when evaluating its progress. The issue of child rights is almost always thought of in terms of exceptional and often criminal abuses; but one of the great breakthroughs made by the Convention is that it specifically rules that malnutrition, preventable disease, and lack of basic education are also violations of children's basic rights. The goals adopted by the World Summit for Children represent a framework for working towards the realization of these rights. And all of the progress documented so far in this report therefore represents practical progress towards the implementation of the Convention on the Rights of the Child.

Stepping-stones

Two points from this brief review of progress since 1990 deserve special emphasis.

First, the achievements recorded here must necessarily be summarized in statistics which are not only inadequate in themselves but convey the scale of what is being achieved only by dehydrating its meaning. Flesh and blood can only be put back by imagining one's own child mentally retarded by iodine deficiency, or crippled for life by polio, or permanently blinded by lack of vitamin A, or stunted in brain and body by malnutrition, or dying from simple, preventable causes like pneumonia, diarrhoea, or measles - and by imagining this tragedy being re-enacted, with all its human nuances, in millions of homes and communities across the world.

Second, these achievements must give pause to those who would take the easy step into cynicism about the value of goals established by the international community. The promises made and the goals adopted at the 1990 Summit have begun to achieve traction in the real world. There have been many important failures and shortfalls. But to a significant degree, the goals established at the World Summit for Children have been and are being translated into reality.

This effort will continue. The 1995 goals are, for the most part, either goals which are easier to achieve or goals which are stages towards the achievement of longer-term and more difficult targets.

But the progress that has been briefly documented here is helping to build the experience and strengthen the outreach systems which will eventually be the means of achieving more difficult and longer-term social development goals.

The industrialized nations

Finally, it is necessary to say a word about the record of the industrialized nations.

They too made their promises at the 1990 World Summit for Children. In addition to re-examining the many problems facing their own children, the industrialized nations promised to review aid programmes with a view to assisting the developing countries to meet the agreed goals. At that time, only a small proportion of all aid - perhaps less than 10% - was being allocated to improvements in nutrition, primary health care, basic education,

Fig. 19 Meeting the mid-decade goals

Number of developing countries on track to achieve the mid-decade goal of reducing the safe water shortfall by one quarter.

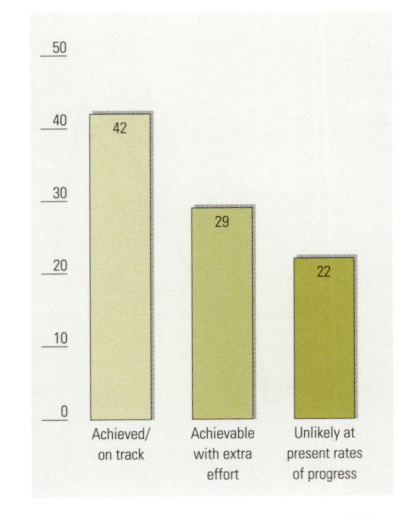

Achieved/on track	Achievable with extra effort	Unlikely at present rates of progress
42	29	22

Source: Country assessments by UNICEF field staff, for 93 countries, September 1994.

Fig. 20 Falling aid levels

Official development assistance (in $ billions at 1992 rates) from the 21 member nations of the OECD Development Assistance Committee.

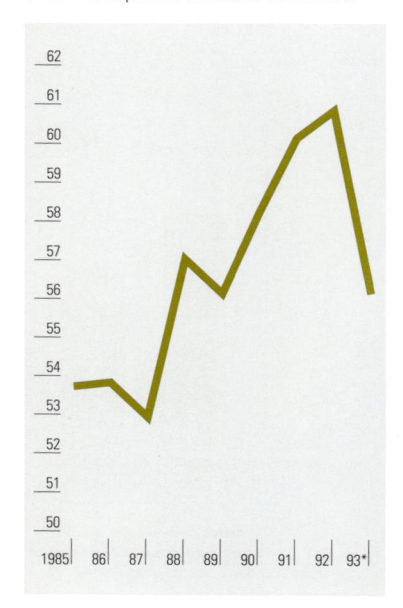

*Provisional figure.

Source: *Organisation for Economic Co-operation and Development, press release, 20 June 1994.*

low-cost water and sanitation services, and family planning (panel 9).

In most industrialized nations, there is little evidence of any significant restructuring of aid in support of the agreed goals.

Instead, we have seen a fall in overall aid levels (fig. 20). Today, the average industrialized nation gives just 0.29% of GNP in aid to the developing world, the lowest for 20 years.[37] Meanwhile, the cost of peace-keeping operations has risen from $0.3 billion to $3.6 billion in the last five years, and the share of United Nations assistance being devoted to relief and emergency work has increased from 25% of the total budget in 1988 to 45% in 1992.[38] These changes may seem insignificant in the larger picture. But any sign of a shift in expenditures from the causes of catastrophe to its consequences should be given a special weight, for it is a sign that the race against time may be being lost.

In some cases, it may be that industrialized countries have held back from commitments in order to see how serious the developing countries themselves were about reaching the agreed goals. In the majority of cases, that question mark has now faded. Formal commitments by the political leaders of the developing world have, in most cases, been followed by significant practical progress. Increased support from the industrialized nations is now essential if this progress is to be maintained, and if the more difficult and expensive year 2000 goals are to be achieved.

There is no valid reason for further delay. Given the political commitment and the practical progress to date, there is now a clear opportunity for the industrialized nations to support this endeavour. The cold war is over; the world of the future faces new and different security threats rooted in poverty and population growth, and environmental deterioration. The progress that has been achieved towards agreed social development goals in the early years of the 1990s, and the much greater progress that could be achieved by the year 2000, attacks some of the root causes of those threats. And support for the developing world's efforts to reach social development goals in the second half of the 1990s is an opportunity to begin building a new post-cold war relationship with the developing world.

Words into deeds   3

SUMMARY: Although specific interventions in such fields as health and nutrition face less resistance than the economic and political changes required to implement today's development consensus, the need now is to identify and build on strategies that work.

The strategies behind the achievements recorded in chapter 2 have included: the breaking down of overall aims into 'doable' propositions; the securing of high-level political support; the mobilization of new social and communications capacities; the deployment of United Nations expertise in close support of agreed goals; and the monitoring and publicizing of progress.

The task facing the World Summit for Social Development is to break down the broader challenges of today's development consensus into doable propositions and to begin mobilizing the necessary support for their achievement. Suggestions for goals have already been put forward by the Secretary-General of the United Nations and by the United Nations Development Programme (UNDP).

Without the specific goals agreed upon at the World Summit for Children the achievements recorded in chapter 2 would not have been possible. But it is equally true to say that the Summit, standing alone, would have achieved relatively little. The crucial factor in translating words into deeds has been the planning, advocacy, and sustained efforts of many tens of thousands of organizations and individuals, both within government and without, who have believed in those goals for children and worked to see them achieved.

This question of implementation, of giving declarations and resolutions some grip and purchase in the real world, is the most important, the most difficult, and the least discussed of all the issues in the development debate. And it is the question which most urgently confronts the World Summit for Social Development. For the real challenge of Copenhagen is not the further refinement and articulation of today's development consensus; it is the finding of practical ways and means to begin translating today's larger development consensus into a larger reality.

And whereas it is undoubtedly true that specific interventions in health and nutrition, however difficult to put into practice on a worldwide scale, face less resistance than the broader changes that will be confronted at the World Summit for Social Development, the need now is to identify and to build on action strategies that work.

This chapter therefore outlines the strategies by which the commitments entered into at the World Summit for Children are being translated into reality.

The principal strategies have been:
☐ the breaking-down of broad goals and objectives into 'doable' and measurable propositions;
☐ the securing and sustaining of the greatest possible political commitment at the highest possible political level - and the simultaneous mobilization of media and public support;
☐ the mobilization of a much wider range of social resources than is conventionally associated with social development efforts - including educational systems, mass media, schools, religious groups, the business com-

munity, and the non-governmental organizations;

☐ the demystification of knowledge and technology in order to empower individuals and families;

☐ the reduction of procedures and techniques to relatively simple and reliable formulas - allowing large-scale operations and the widespread use of large numbers of paraprofessionals;

☐ the deployment of the expertise and resources of the United Nations and its agencies, and of bilateral assistance programmes, in close support of agreed goals. This should include the close monitoring of progress, followed up when necessary by increased support.

Identifying the doable

The selection of goals is crucial to this process.

In theory, goals and target dates should not be necessary for doing what cries out to be done. In practice, such goals are often necessary to translate potential into results: they can make the abstract into the tangible; they can bring a sense of common purpose to the wide variety of organizations and interests that must be involved in any large-scale human enterprise; they can sustain and lend urgency to efforts that are necessarily long term; they can serve as a banner for attracting media attention and public support; they can increase the efficiency of delivery systems; they can introduce the accountability and management by objectives, from the district level up, that are so often the missing cogs in the machinery that links political promises with practical progress.

But there is a crucial distinction to be drawn between a general aim and a specific goal. Overall aims such as 'health for all by the year 2000' sum up a desired end result: goals break down that aim into doable propositions. And it is the doable proposition that has been at the heart of the achievements described in chapter 2 of this report.

In the early 1980s, the task of bringing about major improvements in child health with very limited resources meant that priorities had to be selected. The four priorities adopted by UNICEF were growth monitoring, ORT, breastfeeding, and immunization. These four were chosen because they addressed major specific causes of ill health, poor growth, and early death in almost every developing country; because recent advances in knowledge and technology had made it possible to address these problems at low cost; and because recent advances in social organization and communications capacity had made it possible to make these solutions available on a massive scale. In almost all cases, the solutions were capable of being implemented by following standardized and technically sound guidelines that had already been laid down by WHO. And in each case, the impact of the intervention could be quantified, and progress measured.

As the effort to reach these goals began, universal child immunization emerged as the area where most progress could be achieved.* For this reason, it became a priority among priorities. By the end of 1990, the goal of 80% immunization (75% in sub-Saharan Africa) had been realized in a majority of the developing countries. It has since been reached by many more.

But it also became apparent that immunization could be the thin end of the health wedge. To achieve four or five contacts a year between a modern medical service and over 100 million infants has meant not only building and strengthening outreach systems, but also reorienting health services towards the tasks of reaching out to the unreached, of serving not just those who come through clinic doors but all families in a given area, and of enumerating populations and recording births so that no one is excluded. These are the essential characteristics of a health service that is capable of promoting the wider goals of primary health care. And in many countries today, other health interventions are now being built into these strength-

---

* Originally, the target was universal child immunization by 1990, but when work began to persuade all nations to take this goal seriously, it was clear that if 'universal' were to be interpreted as 100% then the goal was pitched impossibly high. WHO and UNICEF therefore took the realistic decision to redefine the goal to mean that 80% of children should be fully immunized against six major diseases by the age of one year. Ambitious, but not impossible.

There was also much debate at that time over the question of whether striving to achieve specific goals would contribute to or distract from the effort to build primary health care systems: experience has since shown that, in most countries, progress towards particular goals has helped to build the kind of sustainable structures that are necessary for bringing about wider improvements in human health.

ened outreach systems. ORT and vitamin A, for example, are now beginning to reach out to far wider populations than could have been contemplated before the achievement of the 80% immunization goal. In some countries, including India, safe motherhood initiatives and family planning services are also benefiting from the increased outreach capacity that the achievement of the immunization goal has done so much to build.

The process of setting and achieving goals in child health has therefore essentially been one of narrowing down to the doable and then broadening out through the addition of other feasible propositions to what has already been achieved. It is an intensely practical and flexible process, but it is the process by which the overall objective of health for all is most likely to be achieved.

Many other examples could be given. But the essential lesson is that overall aims must first be closely examined to see where the potential breakthroughs can be made. Knowledge, technologies, and the experience that has been gained from 40 years of conscious development efforts must be scrutinized in order to identify the low-cost techniques - whether in health care, water supply, or education - that have been proven to work and are waiting to be put into practice on the same scale as the problems.

Thereafter, it is a case of breaking down overall aims until the doable proposition is identified. Even something as definite as the promotion of breastfeeding is too vague. To become a goal, it must be broken down further into, for example, the 'ten steps' approach and the baby-friendly hospital initiative (see chapter 2). Often, this means setting proxy targets or goals that measure means rather than ends. The elimination of iodine deficiency disorders by the year 2000, for example, needed to be broken down into the even more specific target of iodizing 95% of salt supplies by 1995 before it became a doable proposition.

Time-scale

A goal is not a goal unless it has a date attached and unless progress towards it can be measured. And as most social development goals often have a time-frame of ten years or more, there is a clear danger that target dates will be regarded as being so far in the future that no urgent action is needed. It is therefore also essential to introduce intermediate goals, close monitoring, and periodic reviews of progress.

All of this requires up-to-date and reasonably accurate social statistics. The fact that such statistics are very rarely available is one of the central weaknesses of current social development efforts.

A major strand in today's consensus on development issues is that economic growth alone is no guarantee of human progress, especially for the poorest, and that the universalization of the basic benefits of progress should be both directly promoted and directly measured. Without better statistics, this part of the consensus simply cannot be implemented. The Copenhagen Summit should therefore also attempt to institute new means of generating accurate and timely statistics on all aspects of both social development and social disparity.

As far as possible, monitoring should involve not only political leaders but the media, the non-governmental organizations, and the public. Economic statistics on growth or inflation are today used not only by politicians and economists but by the media and the public in every democratic nation; indeed they are one of the principal means by which politicians are held accountable. If the basic benefits of progress are to be made available to all, then similar use must now begin to be made of annual statistics that record progress, or the lack of it, in nutrition, health care, education, access to health care and family planning, and progress towards equality for women. In sum, social statistics must also become part of the warp and weft of media coverage, of political debate, and of public concern.

Social statistics must become part of the warp and weft of media coverage, of political debate, and of public concern.

Political commitment

Once specific goals have been internationally agreed, high-level political commitment must be mobilized.

In the early 1980s, for example, it was clear that the annual rate of increase in vaccination coverage was not sufficient to carry the world even close to the goal of 80% immunization by 1990. In an attempt to quicken progress, all heads of government in the developing world were asked to make a personal and political commitment to this goal. In 1984 and 1985, over 100 Presidents and Prime Ministers did so. The political mobilization at that time marked the inflection point in immunization's graph: in the second half of the 1980s immunization rates rose rapidly, reaching 80% by the target date of December 1990. During those five years of rapid increase, the majority of the Presidents and Prime Ministers of the developing world were visited by the heads of UNICEF or WHO to appeal for their continued commitment to the achievement of the goal. Many instituted monthly or quarterly reviews of progress, and some participated personally in those reviews. Meanwhile, UNICEF and WHO continued to increase the supply of vaccines, and to assist governments to set up the procedures, establish the cold chains, and overcome the many local and logistical problems. Over the course of the decade, WHO also helped to train thousands of immunization managers and tens of thousands of immunization staff in over 100 countries of the developing world.

The same process has been instrumental in forcing the pace of progress towards the goals adopted at the World Summit for Children.

Following the Summit, UNICEF was charged by the Secretary-General of the United Nations with the task of working with the United Nations family of agencies in order to follow up on the commitments that had been made. That responsibility has so far involved over 100 individual meetings with heads of state. In January of 1994, the Director-General of WHO and the Executive Director of UNICEF also wrote to every head of government in the developing world asking for his or her active leadership in achieving priority social goals by the mid-point in this decade.

Once secured, political commitments must be sustained (and resecured whenever there is a change in government or leadership). The realities of political life mean that the important is constantly under threat from the immediate. Social goals therefore have a tendency to sink without a trace as soon as political waters become choppy - and must be dragged back to the surface at every opportunity.

Wherever possible, the process of building on formal political commitments should begin with the drawing-up of specific national plans for the achievement of agreed goals. In the case of the World Summit for Children, a commitment to national programmes of action (NPAs) was built into the formal resolution by which the goals were adopted. More than 100 nations, with 90% of the developing world's children, have subsequently drawn up NPAs.

Wherever relevant, this process should be repeated at provincial or municipal levels. In the case of the year 2000 goals for children, 50 countries have drawn up subnational plans and 26 more are in the process of doing so. All of China's 22 provinces have prepared their own programmes of action, as have 12 of India's 26 states (covering 85% of its population). In Latin America, 16 of the 24 countries have regional or provincial plans for achieving the goals for children. In Mexico, where every state has its own plan, President Carlos Salinas de Gortari has conducted semi-annual reviews of progress at cabinet level, followed by a nationally televised report. In the Philippines, provincial governors and mayors are committed to local plans of action to reach the goals, and to providing annual progress reports; reviewing these plans, and the progress already achieved,

Following up on the commitments made has so far involved over 100 individual meetings with heads of state.

President Fidel Ramos has declared in 1994: "*Our mid-decade goals are on target. We will finish what we have begun.*"

The limits to what can be achieved by political mobilization of this kind are as clear as the potential benefits: it is not an approach that, on its own, can be expected to bring about fundamental economic change. Yet as part of an overall strategy it has proved its importance. Most analyses of development issues in recent years have led eventually to the point that the political will is lacking to do what could be done. In the future, instead of bemoaning the lack of political will, we must do more to build it.

Social resources

The practical progress that has been made so far towards the year 2000 goals for children has also depended heavily on what has come to be known as the strategy of social mobilization. And it is a strategy which could also help to implement whatever goals emerge from the Copenhagen Summit.

This potential arises from the transformation in social capacity across the developing world. That capacity - to organize, to administer, to reach out to support and inform an entire population - has been transformed by the 2 billion radios and the 900 million television sets that today bring broadcasts, satellite transmissions, and video into most communities. It has been transformed by the rise of literacy to almost 70% and of primary school enrolment to almost 80%, and by the 9,000 daily newspapers and countless numbers of magazines and periodicals that are now being published in the developing world. It has been transformed by the growth of government services, by the more than 5 million doctors and nurses, and the many more millions of community health workers, agricultural extension agents, water and sanitation engineers, trained birth attendants and community development officers who now reach out to the great majority of rural villages and urban neighbourhoods. It has been transformed by the growth of banking and postal services, of electricity, gas and water utilities, of marketing and retailing channels, of the sports and entertainment industries, of the trade union and cooperative movements, of employers' associations and professional societies. And most of all, it has been transformed by the growth of thousands of voluntary agencies, non-governmental organizations, religious societies, people's associations, consumer groups, women's organizations, youth movements, and the millions of local neighbourhood associations, health committees, village councils and their equivalents in almost every country.

The knowledge and the low-cost technologies already exist for the achievement of many of the most obvious goals of social development. Yet too often, the world has remained content with the 'laboratory breakthrough' and failed to also seek the 'social breakthrough' which, in almost all cases, is the vital link between an advance in knowledge and its widespread application.

A vastly greater social capacity now makes it possible to take such knowledge and technologies off the shelf of their potential and to put them at the disposal of the world's families. But this new social capacity for 'going to scale' will remain largely a potential until it is consciously mobilized for social development. Only in the cause of immunization has the potential of social mobilization been realized. And it is significant that immunization remains the only medical breakthrough that has been made available not to 10% or 20% but to the vast majority.

In country after country, the immunization message has gone out via government services and non-governmental organizations, television and radio, newspapers and magazines, churches and mosques, schools and literacy classes, professional bodies and the business community, supermarkets and sports clubs, cinemas and stadiums. Urging on the immunization effort in the late 1980s, WHO Director-

Immunization remains the only medical breakthrough that has been made available not to 10% or 20% but to the vast majority.

General Dr. Hiroshi Nakajima argued:

"We should aim at large-scale mobilization of societal forces for health development ... We must build working alliances with the mass communications sector, with educators in schools, with professional and community organizations, with business, with labour groups and unions. We must break away from our isolation and strive to win partners in our struggle for health promotion." [39]

Today, the potential of social mobilization extends beyond the battleground of health. It can be used to promote and support education and training, family planning and child care, environmental protection and energy efficiency, nutritional improvement and agricultural innovation. It can help to create an informed demand for basic services, and it can help to make available knowledge and technologies for lightening the workloads of women and girls. In all of these areas, inexpensive techniques and technologies already exist. Today's new social capacity could and should be used to put that knowledge at the disposal of every family and every community.

The role of the United Nations

In 50 years of working for development and collaborating with governments and aid agencies in over 150 developing countries, the United Nations family of organizations has built up an enormous fund of experience and expertise in almost every area of social development. This capacity, too, must now be more fully exploited for the implementation of today's development consensus.

In large measure, that development consensus is grounded in the work done by the United Nations and its agencies in the 1970s. The first UN Conference on Human Environment in 1972, the World Population Conference and the World Food Conference in 1974, the UN Conference on Human Settlements in 1976, and, perhaps most significantly, the World Employment Conference of 1976, were major forces in coming to grips with new and complex issues, assessing the trends, and drawing the conclusions that have influenced the world's thinking about these issues over the last 20 years.

But it is true to say that few of the recommendations, goals and targets emerging from these major conferences of the 1970s were translated into widespread programmes of action. Many factors impeded such action. But one of them was that the United Nations had not yet learned how to use its accumulated experience, and its significant operational presence in nearly every country, as a link between internationally agreed goals and practical action on the ground.

Any progress that there might have been in this direction was effectively derailed in the 1980s by the debt crisis, by structural adjustment programmes, by the swing towards an almost exclusive reliance on free-market economic systems, and by a major shift in power towards the Bretton Woods institutions. Much of the work and many of the insights of the 1970s were thereby forgotten.

The swing towards market economic systems was necessary. Command economies had generally failed to meet human needs and prevented people from improving their own lives through their own energies. But whereas it is obvious that free-market economic systems are more capable of generating economic growth, it is far from obvious that they are capable of creating just, civilized, and sustainable human societies. And in the recent commitment to free-market economic policies in many nations of the developing world, supported by the World Bank and the International Monetary Fund, insufficient account has been taken of the effects on the poor, on the vulnerable, or on the environment.

The social and human consequences of this omission are now beginning to be felt. One result is a revival of interest in social development, and this is clearly reflected in the calling of the Copenhagen Summit.

In the recent commitment to free-market economic policies, insufficient account has been taken of the effects on the poor, on the vulnerable, or on the environment.

Not surprisingly, much of the preparation and discussion building up to that Summit links back to the conclusions that were drawn by the United Nations in the 1970s, particularly in its concern over the distribution of economic growth, discrimination against women and girls, and the deterioration of the environment.

Today, there are signs that the United Nations may have begun to develop what was so patently missing in the 1970s - the capacity to make a link between the resolutions of conferences and the practical realization of those plans. The progress that has so far been made towards the year 2000 goals for children, for example, has often depended on close cooperation between UNICEF, other members of the United Nations family, the World Bank, and bilateral assistance agencies. If progress in a particular country has been seen to be faltering, or if monitoring has revealed that current trends are simply not dynamic enough to reach agreed goals, then United Nations agencies and non-governmental organizations have been able to work with governments, often supplying extra personnel and funding, to help bring social development goals back within national sights.

This potential of the United Nations family must now be exploited if the social development goals emerging from Copenhagen are to be translated into action. In so doing, the United Nations can play a key role in responding to new threats to human security in the 21st century - just as it has played a key role in helping to achieve the territorial security of states in the 20th century.

New paradigm

These are the principal strategies by which progress towards the year 2000 goals for children has been achieved. As will be discussed in the next chapter, they cannot, at their present stage of development, bring about change on the necessary scale to implement today's development consensus. But as Dr. Richard Jolly, UNICEF Deputy Executive Director for Programmes since 1982, has said of the strategies discussed here:

"This mixture - which I term a new paradigm for development action - is I believe of widespread applicability. Just as the success of immunization over the 1980s has led on to a broader agenda of goals for improving the health and welfare of children, so this model could also be applied to other areas of international action; to new approaches to peacemaking and conflict prevention; to human development focused on the eradication of poverty; to strengthening of human rights and democratic processes; to environmental protection and sustainable development; to management of global economic and financial relationships. It will require stronger leadership from the international agencies. It will certainly require support from the governments concerned. It will require new means by the United Nations agencies for reaching out to win understanding and support from the publics in individual countries, using the media to explain their mission and to mobilize a greater sense of effectiveness. But above all it will require an abandonment of the cynicism towards international action and some resurgence of hope and belief in the humanitarian mission of the United Nations and of international action more generally. Such vision is not beyond us, and such vision has ... always been present at the most creative periods of the international agencies." [40]

Broader challenges

The task of breaking down the broader challenges of today's development consensus into specific and doable propositions is clearly very much more difficult than anything that has been attempted in the past. And it will require all the expertise that is available in the preparation for, and follow-up to, the World Summit for Social Development.

The commitments entered into at the 1990 World Summit for Children,

Breaking down today's development consensus into doable propositions is very much more difficult than anything attempted in the past.

and the massive effort that has since been made to honour these promises, is an important beginning of a renewed effort to overcome the worst aspects of poverty and slow population growth. The agreement of the great majority of the world's political leaders to a range of specific social development goals in the fields of nutrition, health care, water supply, sanitation, primary education, and family planning has already been made and is, in large measure, being acted on.

A recommitment to those year 2000 goals in Copenhagen is essential if the political and practical momentum behind them is to be maintained.

On the broader front of economic and social development, the Secretary-General of the United Nations has put forward three broad objectives as a basis for discussion in Copenhagen:[41]

☐ the reduction of the proportion of people living in absolute poverty;

☐ the creation of the necessary jobs and sustainable livelihoods;

☐ the significant reduction in disparities among various income classes, sexes, ethnic groups, geographical regions, and nations.

In addition, UNDP has also put forward specific goals for consideration. Its suggestions are:

☐ That the governments of developing countries should allocate at least 20% of their expenditures to meeting priority human needs for adequate nutrition, clean water, safe sanitation, basic health care, primary education, and family planning information and services, and that the industrialized nations should restructure existing aid programmes in order to also allocate a minimum of 20% to these same basic priorities (this is now an agreed position of UNDP, UNICEF, and UNFPA.

☐ That these increases in expenditures on basic social development should be structured into agreements between donor and developing countries designed to meet basic human needs within a defined time - and that progress in implementing these agreements should be internationally monitored.

☐ That both developing and industrialized nations should agree to a targeted annual reduction rate for military spending (UNDP suggests a 3% per year reduction, which would yield approximately $460 billion in the second half of this decade).

The Fourth World Conference on Women, to be held in Beijing in September 1995, could also attempt to break down the overall aim of progress for women into specific goals. Again, the experience gained in recent years should make it possible to advance doable propositions in such fields as equal opportunity legislation, women's reproductive health, equality of educational opportunity, and the widespread promotion of the kind of low-cost technologies that could be an important first step in liberating the time and the energies of many hundreds of millions of rural women in the developing world.

The effectiveness of any and all of these goals will depend upon their being broken down, and if necessary broken down again and again, until the doable propositions are identified. If this can be done, then the Copenhagen Summit will have built the basis for a renewed international development effort in the second half of the 1990s.

Pain now, gain later

4

SUMMARY: More fundamental change is necessary if today's development consensus is to be implemented. In particular, the problems of discrimination, landlessness and unemployment, must be addressed by land reform, investment in small farmers, the restructuring of government expenditures and aid programmes in favour of the poorest, reductions in military expenditures, and significant increases in the resources available for environmentally sustainable development. But the way forward is obstructed by political and economic vested interests, and by the politically unattractive 'pain now, gain later' nature of many of the necessary policies.

The approaches described in the previous chapter have helped to implement significant practical progress in key areas of social development. But this has essentially been a process of taking up the slack of what could be achieved within the status quo. Bringing about more fundamental changes, in the face of the political and economic vested interests that circumscribe the freedom of action of all political leaderships, is a more challenging task.

Yet fundamental change is implicit in today's development consensus. And alongside the effort to identify and achieve doable propositions, there is a need for a simultaneous attempt to push back the boundaries of what is doable. Only by a combination of both processes, the one constantly taking in the slack created by the other, can today's development consensus be translated into reality.

In particular, the problem of the economic marginalization of the poorest nations, and of the poorest people within nations, must be confronted. No social progress can be sustained, no human development can be anticipated, if social and economic exclusion continues to be the chief characteristic of national and global economic systems (fig. 21).

Free-market economic policies have shown that they are successful in the short-term creation of wealth. Governments now have the responsibility to harness that power to the cause of sustainable development. In particular, they have a responsibility to counterbalance the inbuilt tendency of free-market economic systems to favour the already advantaged.

In many developing countries, for example, it is difficult to see how poverty can be overcome without tackling the related issues of discrimination, landlessness, and massive unemployment. In Latin America today, fewer than 10% of landowners own almost 90% of the land.[42] In the Philippines, the proportion of rural workers who are landless has risen from 10% in the 1950s to 50% in the 1990s.[43] In Bangladesh, the poorest 60% of landowners have seen their share of the nation's farm land fall from 25% in 1960 to 10% in 1980. In Africa, which has a reputation for greater equality, it is increasingly the case that most productive lands are devoted to export agriculture while the lands of the poor majority are of lesser quality, receive less investment, and are rapidly becoming degraded and depleted. (The notion that inequality is significantly less in Africa also finds no support whatever from the little information that is available on income distribution: the poorest 20% of the population share only 2.44% of national income in Tanzania, 2.74% in Kenya, and 3.98% in Zimbabwe; in all three of

Fig. 21 Poverty in the developing world
Numbers (in millions) and percentage of population below poverty line in developing countries, 1985 and 1990.

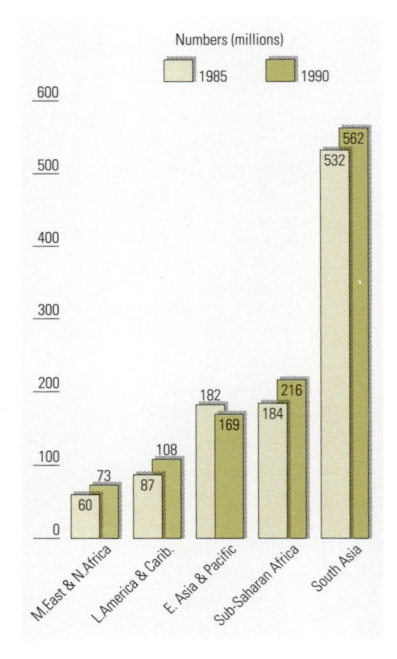

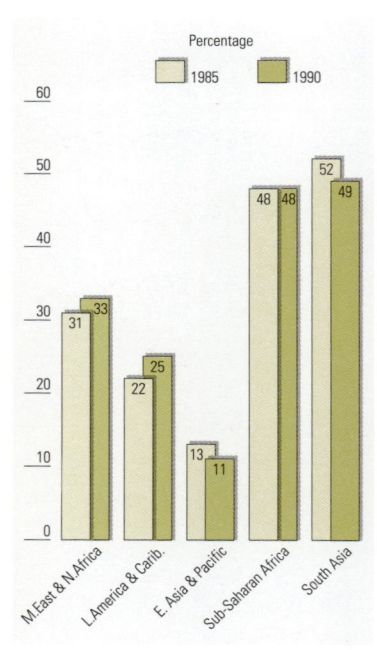

Numbers (millions)
□ 1985 ■ 1990

Region	1985	1990
M.East & N.Africa	60	73
L.America & Carib.	87	108
E. Asia & Pacific	182	169
Sub-Saharan Africa	184	216
South Asia	532	562

Percentage
□ 1985 ■ 1990

Region	1985	1990
M.East & N.Africa	31	33
L.America & Carib.	22	25
E. Asia & Pacific	13	11
Sub-Saharan Africa	48	48
South Asia	52	49

The poverty line is defined here as $31 per person per month at 1985 prices.

Source: World Bank, Implementing the World Bank's strategy to reduce poverty: progress and challenges, 1993. Estimates for 86 countries.

those countries, over 60% of national income accrues to the richest 20% of the people.)[44]

Internationally, inequality has now reached monstrous proportions. Overall, the richest fifth of the world now has about 85% of the world's GNP while the poorest fifth has just 1.4%.[45]

Mark of failure

There are exceptions to this pattern, particularly in South-East Asia: in Indonesia, for example, the proportion of people living below the poverty line has fallen from 60% to 14% in approximately two decades. But in too many nations economic policy is acting as a kind of reverse shock absorber, ensuring that the poor suffer first and most in bad times and gain last and least in good times. Economic development of this kind, whatever the benefits to the better-off, is an economic ratchet which screws the poor ever more tightly to their poverty.

This is no platform for sustained social progress. And the central challenge of development remains the challenge not only of generating environmentally sustainable economic growth but of ensuring that, instead of being marginalized by it, the poor both contribute to it and benefit from it. Only by investing in people and jobs can that challenge be met, as the successful economies of South-East Asia have shown.

Gross inequality - and the rapid population growth which it helps to maintain - mean that large numbers of people are landless, jobless, and incomeless. Add to this poor levels of nutrition, health care, and education, and such people are doubly marginalized, doubly debarred from contributing fully to, or benefiting fully from, the processes of economic and social development.

These are some of the obstacles, buttressed on all sides by powerful vested interests, that must also be overcome if the new challenges to human security are to be met.

Redressing the balance

There is no lack of strategies - or even of broad consensus - for addressing these issues. Of the many proposals that can be feasibly propounded, three or four will serve to illustrate both the possibilities and the difficulties.

☐ Jobs can be created, and productivity by and for the poor can be increased, by policies combining land tenure reform with credit, training, essential infrastructure, the making available of the right technologies to small farmers, and economic policies favouring the use of labour over capital. If this can be achieved, as it has been for example in the South Korea or China (where rural enterprises now employ more than 100 million people and produce more than a third of national output),[46] then the relatively small earnings of very large numbers of people tend to translate into increased demand for better food and health care, better furniture and clothes, better homes and roofs, better tools and small-scale technologies. Much of this demand can be met by local skills and materials, preserving foreign exchange and generating further employment opportunities. By the pursuit of such poor-oriented and labour-intensive patterns of growth, most families could be enabled to meet their own needs.[47] As John Kenneth Galbraith commented in his most recent (1993) contribution to the development debate:

"One of the gravest of past errors has been in associating development with industry, notably primary industry. And farm prices, in frequent cases, have been deliberately kept low as a favour to the urban population. This has been a disastrous error, redeemed too often only in later hunger. It is noteworthy that the developed states, all of them in the past, strongly favoured their farmers and still do ...

"Closely associated with agricultural development is land reform. No country in recent times has flourished under an economic and political system of great landlords or even of small ones. Both economic progress and political democ-

racy require that economic independence be accorded to the men and women who till the land." [48]

An early draft of the declaration that will be made at the Copenhagen Summit acknowledges the point:

"Governments must improve the conditions of the landless poor through land redistribution and land tenure reform, and accompany these with improved access to credit, supplies and equipment, irrigation and water supply systems, markets and extension services. International financial agencies can assist in the process by providing the financial resources needed for land surveys, settlement of conflicting claims and land improvement. The rights of women to hold title to land and to inherit must be ensured and protected." [49]

☐ Government expenditures can be restructured to make major investments in the health, nutrition, and education of the poor. And as many studies have demonstrated, a well-nourished, healthy, and educated population is the most basic investment that can be made in economic and social development.

The case for such restructuring has become a major part of today's consensus on social development.[50] At present, government expenditures in the developing world total approximately $440 billion a year of which only just over 10%, or about $50 billion, is allocated to nutrition, basic health care, primary education, family planning, and clean water and safe sanitation for rural and peri-urban areas.[51] If that proportion were to be increased to 20%, as UNDP, UNFPA, and UNICEF have suggested, then approximately $30 billion a year in extra resources would be made available. In most countries, this would be enough to construct basic social safety nets, and to ensure that minimum human needs were met within a relatively short time.

Most countries could in fact go a long way towards the meeting of basic needs by a fairer allocation of existing social expenditures. In Indonesia, for example, government spending on the health of the richest 10% amounts to three times more than on the poorest 10%.[52] Similarly in India, 75% of government health spending is allocated to curative services in urban areas where 25% of the population lives, and 12,000 medical doctors a year are being trained at the cost of a public whom they do not serve: 80% of graduates go straight into private practice in urban areas.[53]

The same case can be made in education.[54] Most government spending on higher education is spending on the already advantaged: in much of Asia, 50% of government educational spending is devoted to the best-educated 10%; in much of Latin America, more than 50% of government spending on higher education is devoted to the children of families who belong to the richest 20% of the population. The financial cost of achieving primary education for all has been estimated at an extra $3 billion to $6 billion a year: such a sum, representing only about 2% to 3% of the developing world's current annual expenditures on education, could be made available by even a relatively modest restructuring of expenditures away from the better-off and in favour of the poor.

Such distortions are common across the spectrum of basic social services. Of the $10 billion to $12 billion a year that is currently spent on water supply and sanitation, for example, 80% is allocated to relatively high-cost systems - water treatment plants, pumping stations, individual household water supplies, and highly mechanized sewage systems - serving mostly the better-off communities.[55] Meanwhile, only a very small fraction of the available resources is left over for the low-cost community systems that could make clean water and safe sanitation almost universally available at relatively low cost.

Proposals that these expenditure patterns should be shaken up and redirected in favour of the poor are not the product of some radical imagination. The World Bank, for example, has made a significant contribution to this aspect of the current consensus. In its *World Development Report* for 1993, the Bank concluded: *"Governments in*

Government expenditures can be restructured to make major investments in the health, nutrition, and education of the poor.

45

developing countries should spend far less - on average, about 50% less - than they now do on less cost-effective interventions and instead double or triple spending on basic public health programmes."[56] Similarly, on water supply, the Bank argues that government "*can also improve the use of public resources by eliminating widespread subsidies for water and sanitation that benefit the middle class.*"[57]

☐ Similarly, it is a much-repeated part of today's consensus that official development assistance should be restructured in favour of the poor. Only about 25% of today's aid goes to the countries where three quarters of the world's poorest billion people now live. Only about 15% goes to the agricultural sector, which provides a livelihood for the majority of people in almost all developing countries. Only about 2% goes to primary education, roughly 4% to primary health care, and less than 2% to family planning services.[58]

To implement today's development consensus, it will probably be necessary for about 50% of aid and 50% of government expenditures in the developing world to be allocated to a direct attack on poverty. Most of that expenditure should be devoted to the kind of investment that will create jobs and incomes for the poorest fifth of the population. But within that total, 20% of aid and 20% of government expenditures should be devoted to basic social services including nutrition, clean water, safe sanitation, basic health care, primary education, and family planning.

And as almost every commission, report, and conference of the last 20 years has repeated, the industrialized nations should fulfil their pledge to give at least 0.7% of GNP in official development assistance. Currently, only Norway, Sweden, Denmark and the Netherlands are doing so.[59]

☐ Resources can be switched from military capacity to social investment and job creation.

For two decades, military spending in the developing world has grown more than twice as fast as per capita incomes, reaching an annual average of $180 billion throughout the 1980s.[60] This sum is approximately three times as much as the amount that has been received in aid each year, and almost as much as the developing world's annual expenditures on health and education during that decade.[61]

In the 1990s, military spending by most developing countries has fallen. Latest estimates suggest that the current annual total is approximately $120 billion.[62] Yet even this lower sum dwarfs the sums that would be required to provide basic social services. The additional cost of meeting today's unmet demand for family planning, for example, has been put at around $5 billion to $6 billion a year.[63] Similarly, the total cost of achieving universal primary education would be in the region of an extra $3 billion to $6 billion a year. The estimated additional cost of providing clean water and safe sanitation to all communities would be $5 billion to $9 billion a year. And the bill for reaching all of the year 2000 health and nutrition goals would be an additional $11 billion to $13 billion a year.

The money for all of these adds up to about one quarter of the developing world's military expenditures.

And even though military spending is heavily concentrated in the Middle East and parts of Asia, almost all developing countries could finance basic social services by reducing military spending.

The cost of land reforms, infrastructure, training, credit, technology, and of making the essential investments in increased productivity by and for the poor, would require significantly more in the way of government expenditures and foreign aid. But the sums involved are far from impossible. And if it were to be accepted that 50% of government expenditures and 50% of foreign aid programmes were to be devoted to these essential anti-poverty strategies, then it would be possible, within a decade or so, for all countries to achieve the stage of economic development at which not only were basic social services guaranteed but the great majority of today's poor would

Only about 2% of aid goes to primary education, roughly 4% to primary health care, and less than 2% to family planning services.

have the employment by which to meet their own needs by their own efforts.

Vested interests

These are some of the obvious steps that have been suggested as a response to some of the most basic problems of poverty and underdevelopment.

But these central economic problems also point to the central political problem. It has been delicately put by the World Bank. After arguing the case for "*a major redirection of public resources,*" the Bank's 1993 *World Development Report* adds, "*such change will be difficult, since an array of interest groups may stand to lose.*"[64]

In other words, it is salutary to remember the obvious. Such distortions do not happen by accident. The poor remain poor principally because they are underrepresented in political and economic decisions, because their voice is not sufficiently loud in the selection of society's priorities, and because their needs do not weigh sufficiently heavily in the allocation of public resources.

A variant of the same problem faces the attempt to restructure aid programmes. In the United Kingdom, for example, representatives of major companies are asked to advise on the distribution of an aid programme of which they themselves are major beneficiaries in the form of overseas contracts.

All such problems are further compounded by the interlocking nature of vested interests in both donor and recipient countries. And the net result is expenditure patterns which favour the imported over the domestically produced, the capital-intensive over the employment-creating, export crops over local food production, high-cost sewage treatment plants over locally made latrines, household water supply systems over community standpipes, central power stations over fuel-efficient stoves, central teaching hospitals over local health centres, universities over primary schools, the expansion of national airlines over the improvement of local bus services, the construction of the new over the maintenance of the old,[65] industry over agriculture, the military over the social services, the prestigious over the necessary, and ultimately the better-off over the poor.

There will always be powerful vested interests at play in the allocation of public resources. Nor will the forces that have shaped national spending and aid budgets relinquish their hold at the mere appearance of a consensus on what changes should be made. Ultimately, it is democracy itself that must provide the corrective to persistent distortions and injustices. But no democracy, either in the developing world or in the established industrialized nations, has yet achieved this level of sophistication. All democracies have serious flaws and offer imperfect protection against vested interests. Nonetheless, it remains the case that the more effective the democracy the more likely it is, over the long haul, that government policy and government expenditures will reflect the needs of the majority. One of the many reasons why the Indian state of Kerala is such a well-known example of effective health services, low child death rates, low fertility, and near-universal primary and secondary education for girls is that for many decades Kerala, for all its problems and its poverty, has been one of the world's most vibrant democracies (fig. 22).

Despite the set-backs, the march towards democracy across so much of the world in recent years therefore represents the beginning of a change which, if sustained, could fundamentally alter the prospects for development in the decades ahead. But this is a two-way relationship. Democracy makes the sustained achievement of social goals more likely; and social progress makes more likely the survival and development of democracy. As US Secretary of State Warren Christopher has put it, "*the survival of democracies may ultimately depend on their ability to show their citizens that democracy can deliver.*"

The poor remain poor principally because they are underrepresented in political and economic decisions.

After four decades of spending a significant proportion of the world's resources in fighting communism in the name of democracy, the ending of the cold war might logically have been seen as an opportunity to devote an increasing proportion of those resources to social and economic development in those many nations where the shoots of democracy may not long survive because, as yet, they lack the capacity to deliver its fruits.

Asynchronism

The advance and refinement of democracy may be the long-term hope, but the immediate problem must be faced: many if not most of the changes needed to implement today's development consensus run directly counter to deeply entrenched vested interests.

The post-cold war resistance to change by the military-industrial establishment in both industrialized and developing countries is an obvious and formidable example. But in seeking to protect positions of relative privilege, comfort, and security, psychological as well as material, the resistance of the military is not in principle different from the resistance offered by large landholders in relation to the landless, the middle classes in relation to the poor, the industrialized nations in relation to the developing nations, or men in relation to women. For the beneficiaries, all advantages quickly become not unwarranted privileges but expected norms. And most of the people reading this report, as well as most of those involved in its preparation, are in one way or another beneficiaries of privileges from which they would not willingly be separated. The 'better-off' in the developing world - those who would lose by the process of restructuring social expenditures - are for the most part considerably worse off than the great majority of people in the industrialized nations.

The attempt to implement today's consensus also faces a newer problem.

Achieving long-term social goals, meeting minimum human needs, slowing the momentum of population growth, moving towards an environmentally sustainable path of development - all of these suffer from one very obvious disadvantage when it comes to translation into practical policies. For they usually require the kind of measures of which it can be said that the cost must be borne now and the benefits will not accrue until later. And in the case of pre-emptive actions against such threats as global warming or too-rapid population growth, the problem is compounded because the gain is not only long term but takes the form of something that does not happen. It cannot therefore be expected to weigh very heavily in the short-term balance of costs and benefits which is the basis of most political calculation.

There are exceptions to this pattern: the provision of clean water supplies, for example, can offer immediate political rewards as well as immediate health benefits. But generally speaking, the 'pain now, gain later' characteristic of many of the required policies is an enormous handicap. For it is essentially asynchronous with present systems of policy-making. Even in democratic systems, political leaders, with one eye on the opinion polls and the other on the countdown to the next election, have little incentive to pursue policies which incur political or financial costs within their own term of office but deliver their benefits only to future generations. Similarly, the business and commercial world normally operates within relatively short timeframes for the securing of returns on investment. It, too, is therefore unlikely to show a sustained interest in initiatives tagged with the 'pain now, gain later' label.

This problem of asynchronism between the time-frame of the required policies and the time-frame of most policy makers represents a serious challenge to the capacity of modern political systems to cope with the world's mounting long-term problems. It is a problem which can only become more acute, and any fundamental resolution will require nothing less than the development of more sophisticated

Many of the changes needed to implement today's development consensus run directly counter to deeply entrenched vested interests.

Fig. 22 Kerala factor

In wealth, the Indian state of Kerala falls below the average for India as a whole. In social progress it is considerably more advanced. Along with Kerala's long history of progressive social policies, two of the most powerful factors are a tradition of participatory democracy and a strong commitment to female education. Almost all girls complete secondary as well as primary education.

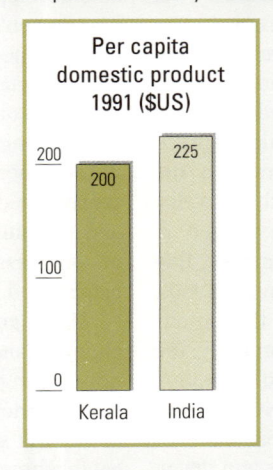

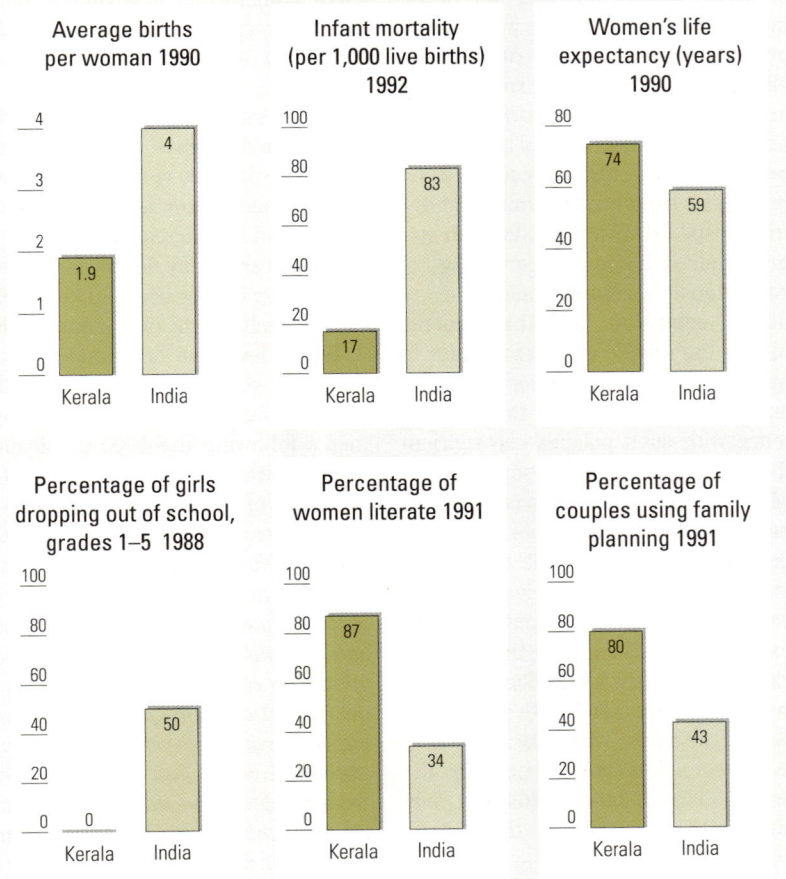

Per capita domestic product 1991 ($US)
- Kerala: 200
- India: 225

Average births per woman 1990
- Kerala: 1.9
- India: 4

Infant mortality (per 1,000 live births) 1992
- Kerala: 17
- India: 83

Women's life expectancy (years) 1990
- Kerala: 74
- India: 59

Percentage of girls dropping out of school, grades 1–5 1988
- Kerala: 0
- India: 50

Percentage of women literate 1991
- Kerala: 87
- India: 34

Percentage of couples using family planning 1991
- Kerala: 80
- India: 43

Source: Government data, chiefly from sample registration system and 1991 census,

One of the reasons why Kerala is such a well-known example of low child death rates, low fertility, and near-universal education is the vibrancy of its democracy.

democracies and the evolution of a more informed and involved public.

Creeping change

To a limited extent, these two fundamental and related problems - of vested interest and asynchronism - can be circumvented by approaches based on gradual and incremental change. Targets can be set for reductions in military expenditures which spread the pain over many years into the future. The criteria on which aid is allocated can gradually be changed in favour of the poor in the same way that they have been changed, in the 1990s, to favour democracy and the protection of the environment. Similarly, the restructuring of health and education budgets can be achieved over a period of time by limiting future expenditures on universities or hospitals and devoting the greater part of any increases to primary schools and to rural health clinics. Zimbabwe, for example, has imposed a ten-year moratorium on any new investments in central hospitals in order to concentrate resources on improving rural health clinics and district hospitals.[66] Similarly, India is progressively reducing the percentage of educational spending allocated to higher education (and that benefits mainly the middle classes) in order to move towards at least basic education and literacy for all. Over time, persistence with such policies can reorient the allocation of resources: in Malaysia, health policy has been oriented towards the poor for two decades, with the result that lower income groups now receive a considerably greater share of public health expenditures than do the middle classes. Similarly, Costa Rica has pursued a poor-oriented health policy over several decades, with 30% of government spending now benefiting the poorest 20% of households and only 10% being allocated to the richest 10%.[67]

But in the great majority of the world's countries, a large question mark must remain over whether such incremental approaches are likely to be introduced or whether they are capable of bringing about changes as fundamental as those now required - including reductions in military expenditures, increases in the resources available for environmentally sustainable development, the restructuring of government expenditures and of aid programmes, the ending of discrimination against women and girls, the reduction of fertility through both family planning services and the kind of improvements in people's lives that create the desire for smaller families, and a rethink of the unsustainable path of progress being pursued in the established industrialized countries.

These are radical and far-reaching changes, and they have been called for not by fringe groups or voices crying in the wilderness but by commissions or reports set up by the international establishment and involving some of the most eminent and experienced statesmen and stateswomen of our times.

Yet it cannot be denied that after years of such reports, and the constant repetition of such appeals, the action that has been taken is in no way adequate. And an increasing number of observers are today despairing, and in some cases frankly scornful, of the efficacy of such efforts and such appeals.

Such views can be summed up in the blunt assessment of one of the experts invited to contribute comments following the 1990 publication of the South Commission's report *The Challenge to the South*:

"I believe myself that the next 20 years of North-South negotiations are not going to be more significant or efficacious than the last 20 years.... An appeal of the liberals among the powerful to their compeers to make reforms in the interest of equity, justice, and heading off worse has never had any significant effect in the past several hundred years except in the wake of direct and violent rumblings by the oppressed, and it will have no more effect now."[68]

The voice of many contemporary critics is represented here. And the answer to the question it poses - the

After years of reports and appeals, an increasing number of observers are despairing of the efficacy of such efforts.

question of whether the changes called for by today's consensus on development issues are too radical and too far-reaching to have any chance of being put into practice on the necessary scale and in the face of prevailing vested interests - will determine success or failure in the attempt to make the transition to a sustainable human future.

On the basis of history alone, such a view can be challenged. It is simply not true that, over the last several hundred years, reports and commissions and appeals have proved incapable of achieving change in the direction of equity, justice and *"heading off worse."* The process of argument and debate, and appeals to reason, conscience, and enlightened self-interest, have played a major part in the struggle against racism, colonialism, apartheid, and in the progress made over recent decades towards equality for women. And whereas it is true that the *"direct and violent rumblings of the oppressed"* have always been counted among the principal causes of change, it is also true that fundamental change has many times been brought about not by violence and revolution but by democratic political processes that have framed an intelligent and far-sighted response to the problems of poverty and oppression. Not to accept this is to imply that rapid and fundamental change can only come about through a revolutionary rejection of the status quo and all its institutions. That view, long sincerely held by many who believed passionately in justice, is today considerably the less attractive for having been tried. Invariably, the result has been the concentration of power into even fewer hands and the entrenching of unaccountable regimes that have failed either to respect basic human rights or to meet basic human needs.

As for the possibilities for change in the near future, the final chapter of this report puts forward the case against pessimism. New and enormously powerful forces for change are now at work in the world. And they are changing the rules of the game of change itself.

5 Unfinished business of the 20th century

SUMMARY: The effort to achieve social development goals is part of a historic struggle to restructure societies in the interests of the many rather than the few. Only in this century has that ideal begun to make significant practical headway. Combined with the continuing increase in worldwide productive capacity that began with the industrial revolution, this change in the underlying social ethic has made it possible to put the basic benefits of progress at the disposal of all. Completing this revolution is the unfinished business of the 20th century.

The successes that have been achieved so far in this struggle have not been brought about by any inevitable force of history or technology, but by a conscious effort - led less by governments than by people - to make morality march with advancing capacity. The involvement of even larger numbers of people in this struggle is the best hope for fundamental change, for implementing today's development consensus, and for bringing what must be done within the bounds of what can be done.

The effort to advance social development, and to make the most basic benefits of progress available to all, is a cause which, in various forms, has inspired men and women throughout the ages. But it is a cause which has only begun to gain significant traction in this century. And it is this historical context which is the strongest argument against pessimism.

For ten thousand years, civil societies have almost invariably been structured by, and for the principal benefit of, a small proportion of their members. And for most of those ten thousand years, this state of affairs has been promoted as normal, natural, and necessary. Codifying this tendency in a famous book, the 19th-century Italian scholar Gaetano Mosca noted:

"Among the constant facts and tendencies that are to be found in all political organisms, one is so obvious that it is apparent to the most casual eye. In all societies, two classes of people appear - a class that rules and a class that is ruled. The first class - always the less numerous - performs all political functions, monopolizes power and enjoys the advantages that power brings, whereas the second, the more numerous class, is directed and controlled by the first, in a manner that is now more or less legal, now more or less arbitrary and violent." [69]

Only against the background of the astonishing geographical and historical durability of these *"constant facts and tendencies"* can the scale of this century's achievements be seen.

Almost every previous era, for example, would have found absurd, if not treasonous, the notion that society should be organized in the interests of the many, or that the benefits of knowledge should be shared by all. In ancient Egypt, in pre-colonial India, and in Europe from the days of the Druids to the end of the Middle Ages, the written language, and access to religious texts, were deliberately restricted in order to preserve the status and power of the few.

Until comparatively recent times, that power has never been allowed to travel very far from the centre of any society. Even the celebrated direct democracy of 5th-century Athens was a government of the few, by the few, for the few, with no place and no vote for women, for manual labourers, for free men without sufficient property, or for the 60,000 - 80,000 slaves and chattels who tended the cradle of democracy. Almost 2,000 years later, in the new Athens of Renaissance Florence, power and privilege were also concentrated, except for the briefest of periods, in the hands of 150 families whose combined wealth exceeded that of 90% of the Florentine citizenry: only those of "*status and substance*" could hold office, and they did so "*for the benefit of the rich and powerful at the expense of the poor and lowly.*"[70] Similarly, in the France of the Enlightenment, the idea that the mass of the people existed to serve the state and its élite was reflected in legislation that specifically exempted the land-owning nobility from taxes but forced those who tilled the land to pay more than a quarter of their incomes to finance the wars, the pageants, and the châteaux of the state.[71]

Divine sanction

Such extremes of élitism were maintained not only by force but by an underlying ethic which sought to present this state of affairs as divinely approved. China's mandarins justified their exclusive rule on the basis that they alone could interpret the will of the gods; Islamic leaders have sometimes invoked the same principle to justify the exclusion of the people from participation in government; and long before the British raj attempted to authenticate its rule in India with the stamp of duty and religion, Hindu élites had refined their own methods of ensuring that the lower orders knew their place.

Even when in direct contradiction to the most basic teachings of religion, such class divisions have insisted on their divine legitimacy. The Christian message, for example, has often been corrupted to serve the "*rich and powerful at the expense of the poor and lowly*" and to let the latter know that their inferior status was ordained by God: in Sunday schools and churches throughout the Christian world today, a favourite hymn continues to remind the faithful that "*The rich man in his castle, the poor man at his gate, God gave them all their station, and ordered their estate.*"[72]

This idea of a class born to rule, and to enjoy thereby a virtual monopoly of privilege and progress, has survived in one form or another - aristocrat over peasant, white race over black, European over Asian and African, owner over worker, male over female - even through the great liberal revolutions of the modern era. The American Revolution of 1776 left slavery intact. The French Revolution of 1789 resulted not only in dictatorship but, as Marat complained in the 1790s, in the replacement of an aristocracy of birth by an aristocracy of wealth. And in the following century, the independence movements of Latin America brought to power governments which, in the words of historian Emilia Viotti da Costa, "*took no account of the mass of the population, whom they feared and despised.*"[73] Similarly, 20th-century struggles against colonialism in Africa and Asia have often resulted, as Rajni Kothari has written, "*in no more than a transfer of power from one élite to another.*"[74]

Unfinished business

Only in this century, and particularly in the last 50 years, have these "*constant facts and tendencies*" begun to be transformed.

Half a century ago, over 50 nations in Africa and Asia were ruled from London, Paris, Lisbon, Brussels, or The Hague. Half a century ago, the National Party was about to introduce formal apartheid in South Africa. Half a century ago, communism, which had substituted the party for the class that was born to rule, was establishing itself across Eastern Europe and beginning its advance into many areas of the developing world. Half a century ago, women in France and Japan did

Half a century ago, over 50 nations in Africa and Asia were ruled from London, Paris, Lisbon, Brussels, or The Hague.

The underlying ethic that has endured for so much of human history is clearly losing its grip on human affairs.

not have the right to vote. And half a century ago, across much of the United States, a black person could neither vote, nor serve on a jury, nor eat in certain restaurants, nor occupy a bus seat if a white person was standing.

As an overall indication of this change, it need only be noted that 50 years ago only a small proportion of the world's people had a voice or a vote in the selection of those who governed them; today, the proportion has risen to between half and three quarters.

Many societies are still divided into unaccountable rulers and unconsenting ruled. Many more remain divided into privileged few and impoverished many. In most, the basic benefits of progress have not yet been made available to the majority. Nonetheless, one would have to be not just a cynic but a recluse to deny that this age-old order is being shaken in our times. At a minimum, the underlying ethic that has endured for so much of human history is clearly losing its grip on human affairs; there is hardly a society in the world today where the idea of a class that is born to rule, an idea defended by moral philosophers and political leaders from Aristotle to Churchill, is accepted as right, or normal, or in the nature of things'.

Nor has this change been confined to breakthroughs in principle. Made possible by a massive and continuing increase in world productive capacity, the idea that the aim of progress, and of government, is to benefit the majority of the people has, in the second half of this century, brought enormous practical change (fig. 23). Average life expectancy in the developing nations - that useful composite measure of improvements in incomes and nutrition, health care and education - has increased from approximately 40 years in 1950 to 62 years by 1990. Child death rates have fallen by two thirds, from around 300 to 100 per 1,000 births. Adult literacy rates have doubled to almost 70%. Smallpox, which killed approximately 5 million people a year in the early 1950s, has been eradicated. Polio, measles, malnutrition, micronutrient deficiencies, and diarrhoeal disease are being beaten. Overall, concluded the World Bank in 1993, "*health conditions across the world have improved more in the past 40 years than in all of previous human history.*"[75]

These achievements were but a vision when the United Nations was founded. In 1952, the United Nations *Report on the World Social Situation* heralded the "*historical and inspiring fact*" that the world was being made one, and endorsed the hope of the historian Arnold Toynbee that "*the 20th century will be chiefly remembered in future centuries not as an age of political conflicts or technical inventions, but as an age in which human society dared to think of the welfare of the whole human race as a practical objective.*"[76] Difficult as it may be to imagine from the day-to-day headlines, a longer-term view shows that the last 50 years have done much to justify this prophecy.

Sea change

This is the historical context of the struggle for development that is now reaching such a critical stage. And the particulars of that struggle - including the setting of goals for the protection of children and the attempt to bring such services as immunization, basic health care, family planning, water and sanitation, or primary education to all communities - are part of the attempt to carry this struggle through to its completion. They are the manifestation of the idea that the most basic advantages of progress should be put at the disposal of all; and they are the embodiment of the principle that society should be organized in the interests of the many rather than the few.

Completing this historic process is the chief unfinished business of the 20th century. And on our success or failure will depend the outcome of the race against time. Only if this cause is seen through to a conclusion in the years immediately ahead will it be possible for the world to cope with the problems of population growth, envi-

Fig. 23 Progress in basics

The effort to make the most basic benefits of progress available to all has achieved remarkable results in the half-century since the founding of the United Nations. Few reliable statistics are available from the 1940s, but the charts below summarize the progress that has been made in the three decades from 1960 to 1990.

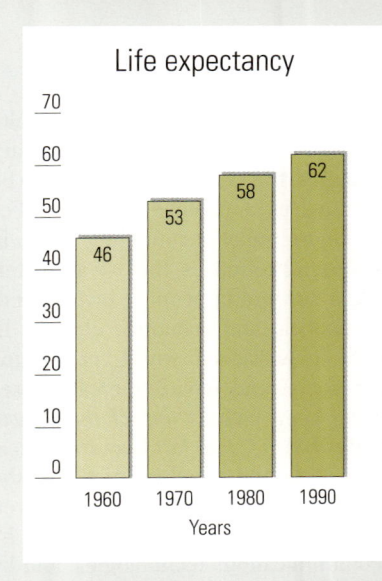

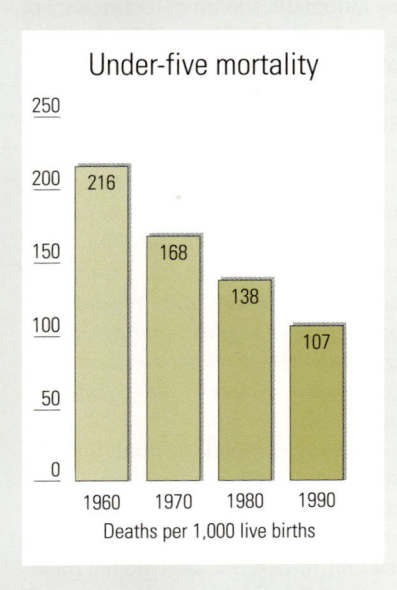

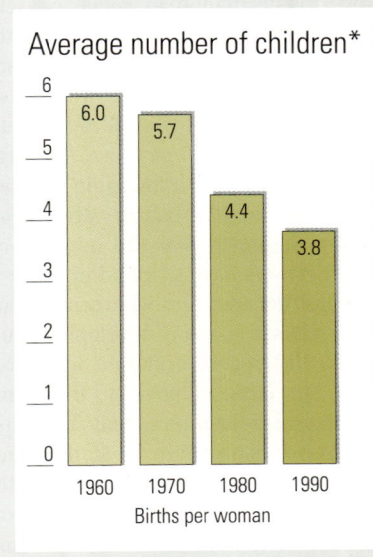

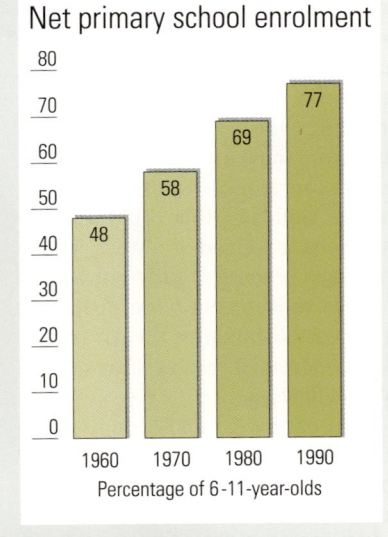

Life expectancy
(Years)
- 1960: 46
- 1970: 53
- 1980: 58
- 1990: 62

Under-five mortality
(Deaths per 1,000 live births)
- 1960: 216
- 1970: 168
- 1980: 138
- 1990: 107

Average number of children*
(Births per woman)
- 1960: 6.0
- 1970: 5.7
- 1980: 4.4
- 1990: 3.8

Net primary school enrolment
(Percentage of 6-11-year-olds)
- 1960: 48
- 1970: 58
- 1980: 69
- 1990: 77

*The figures given are for the total fertility rate — the number of children that would be born per woman if she were to live to the end of her child-bearing years and bear children at each age in accordance with prevailing age-specific fertility rates.

Sources: *Life expectancy and fertility:* UN Population Division, World population prospects: the 1992 revision, *1993; under-five mortality:* UNICEF; *school enrolment:* UNESCO, Trends and projections of enrolment by level of education, by age and by sex, 1960–2025, *1993*.

Health conditions across the world have improved more in the past 40 years than in all of previous human history.

It is the power of concerned and committed people, and their organizations, that can bring what needs to be done within the bounds of what can be done.

ronmental deterioration, social disintegration - and the challenge of sustaining new democracies (panel 10).

The history of this struggle also teaches the one all-important lesson for the battles that still lie ahead. For the successes that have been achieved so far have not been brought about by any automatic spread of technology or by any inevitable force of history. They have been brought about by a conscious effort to make morality march with capacity. As Martin Luther King said of the civil rights struggle:

"Human progress is neither automatic nor inevitable. Even a superficial look at history reveals that no social advance rolls in on the wheels of inevitability. Every step towards the goals of justice requires sacrifice, suffering, and the tireless exertions and passionate concern of dedicated individuals." [77]

No heavier weight of tradition, and no more deeply entrenched vested interests, for example, have ever been arrayed against progress than those that confronted the anticolonial movements of this century or the women's movement and the environmental movement of 30 years ago. Yet the very idea of imperialism, once revered, has been rendered unacceptable. Similarly, the environmental and women's movements have made progress - progress in attitudes, policy, practice, and law - that could scarcely have been imagined at a time, so few years ago, when the early supporters of those movements were dismissed by the establishment of the day as misguided extremists on the fringe of the political dialogue.

No progress is rapid enough in the face of injustice and discrimination, or when the physical integrity of the biosphere is under threat. But by any historical standards, changes in attitude and actions in these two areas have been both profound and extraordinarily rapid. And they have been brought about less by governments than by people's movements, by a people-led sea change in public perceptions of what is and is not acceptable in human affairs - and by a corresponding change in the perceptions of democratic political leaders as to what constitutes good politics. And as these examples show, it is above all the power of concerned and committed people, and their organizations, that can bring what needs to be done within the bounds of what can be done.

New forces for change

If this is indeed the force that can ultimately bring about the necessary changes, then the balance may now be shifting in a positive direction. For there are today encouraging signs, in almost all countries, that we are entering a new era of people's involvement in political and economic change. In the industrialized world, campaigns for social and environmental causes have been called *"one of the growth industries of the late twentieth century."*[78] In the developing world, the rise of such movements has been even more extraordinary: stimulated by communications technologies, and by the transformation in social capacity that has already been discussed, the number of people's movements and non-governmental organizations has risen rapidly in almost all developing countries over recent years. Although this movement is impossible to quantify, even the most conservative of estimates suggests that the numbers of such groups have doubled or more in the last decade. And whereas the surface signs in so many developing countries, the macroeconomic indicators and the facts of poverty, debt, and structural adjustment, may be cause for pessimism, there is at the same time a great cause for hope in the emergence at the micro-level of thousands of groups and organizations, whether their reach is the neighbourhood or the nation, that are working for change.

This growth of people's involvement in the struggle for change has deep roots. It is rooted in the dramatic increase in productive capacity which has opened up an unprecedentedly wide gap between the world as it is and the world as it could be. And it is rooted in the equally spectacular increase in communications capacity which has made that gap more visible to more people than ever before. In recent years, communications technologies have spread an awareness of the modern world, its possibilities and its choices, to every community on the globe, provoking the comparisons, allowing the judgements, changing the attitudes, heightening frustrations, holding out visions, creating a new capacity for people to communicate with one another, and fermenting the brew of change. In almost all countries today, the contours of the possible are being reshaped as people find a new solidarity and a new confidence in their own rights and abilities to participate in the management of their own affairs. No longer are people willing to accept that societies should be so organized that progress, knowledge, and rights, should remain the monopoly of the few.

There will be those who doubt whether anything so amorphous can be a major force for change. But in the 1990s, they must ask themselves why it is that revolutionary changes have been achieved in Latin America, in South Africa, in Central and Eastern Europe, and in the countries of the former Soviet Union, over so little time and with so little transitional violence. They must ask themselves, for example, how likely it would have seemed ten years ago that the Berlin Wall would soon fall and that the cold war would suddenly come to an end. And they might ask themselves, also, how realistic it would have seemed that, within far less than a decade, President Lech Walesa would be sending a telegram of congratulation to President Nelson Mandela.

In the past, such stirrings for change have often been met with repression. But in several recent and prominent instances, representatives of the old order have realized that repression is becoming a less and less attractive option. And again, it is the power of communications that has meant that oppressive regimes are no longer quite so free to act arbitrarily, or in secrecy, or with impunity, against isolated, inarticulate, unorganized, and unsupported peoples.

Finally, it should not be ignored that new pressures for change are also beginning to emerge from within the industrialized world. In almost all of the economically developed nations, there is a palpable and increasing anxiety about the current trajectory of progress - even in the ranks of those who could be said to be among its principal beneficiaries. Faith in such progress, so evident in the 1950s and 1960s, has been jolted in the last decade or so by two forces. The first is a spreading realization that current patterns of consumption and pollution are environmentally unsustainable. The second is a widespread perception that such progress is also failing to bring with it significant further improvements in the quality of life for large numbers of people. The established industrialized nations, that small group of the most affluent societies the world has ever seen, are societies where absolute poverty remains a problem, where evident unhappiness is common even among the relatively well-off, and where social and environmental problems, from crime to family breakdown, from mental illness to drug abuse, from pollution to mental stress, are all perceived to be increasing. *"The look into the future which was once tied to a vision of linear progress,"* as Susan Sontag has written, is becoming instead *"a vision of disaster."*[79]

In the face of all of such forces, building up inexorably as the 20th century comes to an end, the possibilities for bringing about fundamental changes, so often called for and so often ignored, are therefore no longer remote. Inasmuch as anything in the future is ever clear to the present, it is clear that fundamental change is at hand.

Common cause

Diversity and passionate commitment to a thousand individual causes -

No longer are people willing to accept that societies should be so organized that progress, knowledge, and rights, should remain the monopoly of the few.

Panel 10

The PPE spiral: and the new security crisis

Last year's *State of the World's Children* report discussed the interaction between poverty, population growth, and environmental deterioration. To stress the inseparable nature of these problems, the report used the term 'PPE problem'. This year's report stresses that the new generation of security threats arises in large part from the synergisms between PPE problems and social and political instabilities. The diagram schematizes the argument.

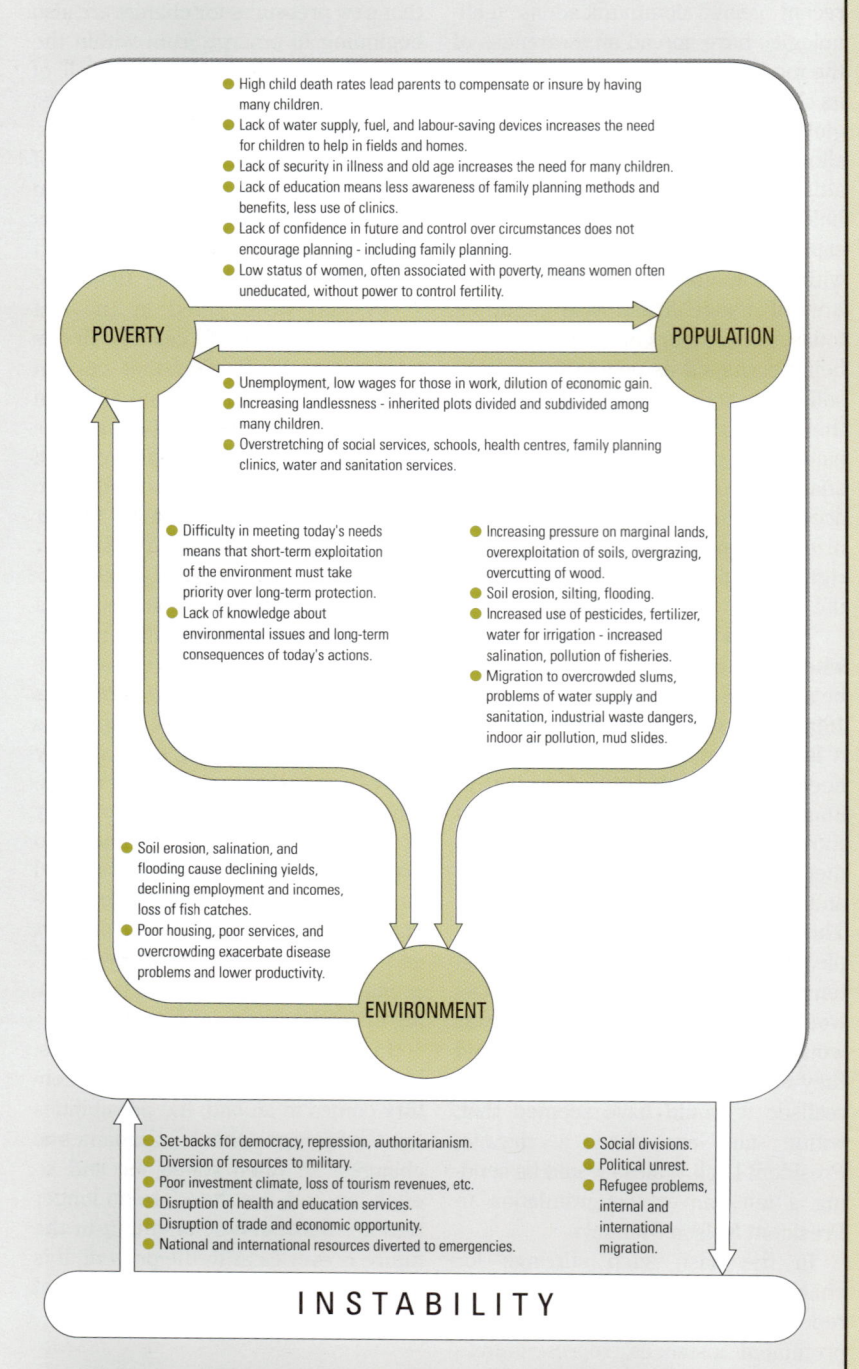

POVERTY → POPULATION

- High child death rates lead parents to compensate or insure by having many children.
- Lack of water supply, fuel, and labour-saving devices increases the need for children to help in fields and homes.
- Lack of security in illness and old age increases the need for many children.
- Lack of education means less awareness of family planning methods and benefits, less use of clinics.
- Lack of confidence in future and control over circumstances does not encourage planning - including family planning.
- Low status of women, often associated with poverty, means women often uneducated, without power to control fertility.

POPULATION → POVERTY

- Unemployment, low wages for those in work, dilution of economic gain.
- Increasing landlessness - inherited plots divided and subdivided among many children.
- Overstretching of social services, schools, health centres, family planning clinics, water and sanitation services.

POVERTY → ENVIRONMENT

- Difficulty in meeting today's needs means that short-term exploitation of the environment must take priority over long-term protection.
- Lack of knowledge about environmental issues and long-term consequences of today's actions.

POPULATION → ENVIRONMENT

- Increasing pressure on marginal lands, overexploitation of soils, overgrazing, overcutting of wood.
- Soil erosion, silting, flooding.
- Increased use of pesticides, fertilizer, water for irrigation - increased salination, pollution of fisheries.
- Migration to overcrowded slums, problems of water supply and sanitation, industrial waste dangers, indoor air pollution, mud slides.

ENVIRONMENT → POVERTY

- Soil erosion, salination, and flooding cause declining yields, declining employment and incomes, loss of fish catches.
- Poor housing, poor services, and overcrowding exacerbate disease problems and lower productivity.

ENVIRONMENT

INSTABILITY

- Set-backs for democracy, repression, authoritarianism.
- Diversion of resources to military.
- Poor investment climate, loss of tourism revenues, etc.
- Disruption of health and education services.
- Disruption of trade and economic opportunity.
- National and international resources diverted to emergencies.
- Social divisions.
- Political unrest.
- Refugee problems, internal and international migration.

The above chart is limited to processes within the developing world. But the PPE spiral is compounded by the industrialized world's policies in the fields of aid, trade, finance, and debt.

whether it be the AIDS crisis or the preservation of local environments or the safeguarding of forests or the protection of women from violence - is the hallmark of the current upsurge in people's movements that is the chief hope for the future. But if it is to be people's involvement that changes the prevailing ethical climate, and makes possible the transition to a sustainable future, then it is essential that those movements also now come to a common focus on some of the basic problems underlying their ostensibly different concerns.

Above all, it is essential that the needs and the rights of children should become the common cause and common cry of action groups and people's movements the world over. Protecting and investing in the physical, mental, and emotional development of all children is the foundation of a better future, the end and the means of development, the very foundation for economic development, social cohesion, and political stability. And unless this investment is made, all of humanity's most fundamental long-term problems will remain fundamental long-term problems.

Whatever the particular cause, be it democracy or human rights, development or equity, gender equality or environmental protection, the growth, development, and education of children is central to long-term success.

Starting with the basic and specific goals of survival, health, and education that have already been accepted by the international community, the cause of children must now be taken up by the thousands of groups and the millions of people who are now becoming involved in working for change, in so many different ways, for so many particular causes, and in almost all the countries of the world.

In the past, many may have been dissuaded from this struggle by its apparent hopelessness, by the idea that meeting the basic needs of all children is too difficult, too vast and too expensive a task to be achieved in the immediate future. And one of the great tasks of the people and organizations working for this cause is to dispel these myths.

The principal technologies for meeting children's needs at relatively low cost are already available. The social capacity is largely in place. And the financial cost is frankly negligible in relation to what humanity has at stake in this race. It has been estimated by UNDP, UNFPA, and UNICEF, for example, that the total cost of providing basic social services in the developing countries, including health, education, family planning, clean water, and all of the other basic social goals agreed on at the World Summit for Children, would be in the region of an additional $30 billion to $40 billion a year, two thirds of which could come from the developing countries themselves. The world spends more than this on playing golf.[80] The United States share of this bill would be less than is spent, nationally, on advertising tobacco. The private sector has been known to mobilize $30 billion for a single major construction project - a dam, a tunnel, an airport. Governments find such sums as a matter of course: the United States spends $25 billion a year on its prison service alone;[81] Germany finds more than $30 billion each year to meet the social costs of reunification; Japan is about to invest approximately ten times as much in an optical fibre network for the next century.[82]

Meeting children's needs depends not just on social services but on their parents having jobs and incomes. The cost of a major effort to bring about land reforms, invest in small producers, and create large numbers of jobs would be very much more than $30 billion a year. Double it; it is still less than the world spends on wine.[83] Triple it; it is still far less than the world spends on cigarettes.[84]

Even if the resources were to be made available, money alone is not sufficient. Sustained political commitment and competent management are just as important. But to say that the world cannot at this stage afford the financial cost of meeting its children's needs and ending some of the very

Unless the investment in children is made, all of humanity's most fundamental long-term problems will remain fundamental long-term problems.

59

Where there have been thousands of organizations there must be tens of thousands, where there have been tens of thousands of people, there must be millions.

worst aspects of poverty, malnutrition, preventable disease, and illiteracy, is plainly absurd. And there is a need to kindle a new sense of this absurdity among a worldwide public. Of course the normal growth and development of children can be protected. Of course absolute poverty can be overcome. Of course population growth can be slowed. Of course environmental deterioration can be arrested. For decades now, this has not been a question of possibilities but of priorities. And the truth of the matter is that these problems could and should have been largely defeated in the 1970s and 1980s: if one tenth of the resources that have been devoted to building military capacity over those decades had been devoted to achieving basic development goals, then we would now be living in a world with little or no malnutrition, with far less disease and disability, with far higher levels of literacy and education, with higher incomes and lower birth rates, with fewer social and environmental problems, with fewer civil conflicts and refugees, and with fewer and less destructive wars.

This comparison between military expenditures and human needs may be the most often repeated cliché in the development dictionary. But we must never tire of making it, never allow this state of affairs to be countenanced as in any way civilized or justifiable, never allow the most blatant imbalance of our times to subside into the tacitly accepted. Even in the post-cold war era, the world annual expenditure on military capacity, on missiles, tanks, aircraft, fighter planes, remains at a level that is *four times the combined annual incomes* of the poorest quarter of the developing world's people - the 1 billion absolute poor, those who are without the basics of life, those without education and jobs, those without clean water or basic health care, those whose children die and become disabled in such numbers, those who are forced to ruin their own environments and futures for the sake of staying alive today.

Becoming involved

A people-led change in the climate of ideas, in what is considered acceptable or unacceptable in the relationships between people and nations, is the best hope that the great changes to come will be changes for the better. The common focus of that effort must be to give the protection of the normal physical, mental, and emotional development of children a first call on our concerns and capacities. And a first step towards that aim is to achieve the basic goals for the world's children that have already been established and behind which considerable momentum has already been built.

But if the race against time is to be won, then where there have been thousands of organizations there must be tens of thousands, where there have been tens of thousands of people, there must be many millions.

And by becoming involved in this struggle, in whatever way and on whatever front, it may be that an answer will also be found to the problems which today beset so many of those, in all nations of the world, who are the principal beneficiaries of the progress that has been achieved in this century. For it may be that the being involved in a cause larger than oneself is a deep human need from which we have been diverted by the particular direction that progress has taken in recent times. If so, it is a need of which George Bernard Shaw has left us a powerful reminder:

"This is the true joy in life, the being used for a purpose recognized by yourself as a mighty one. I am of the opinion that my life belongs to the whole community and as long as I live it is my privilege to do for it whatever I can. Life is no brief candle to me. It is a sort of splendid torch which I have got hold of for the moment, and I want to make it burn as brightly as possible before handing it on to future generations." [85] ☐

REFERENCES

1. United Nations Development Programme, *Human Development Report 1994*, UNDP, New York, 1994, fig. 4.3, p. 63
2. World Bank, *World Development Report 1994: Infrastructure for Development*, World Bank, Washington, D.C., 1994, table 30, p. 220
3. Johnson, Clifford M., and others, *Child Poverty in America*, Children's Defense Fund, Washington, D.C. 1991
4. United Nations, Department of Public Information, 'The Job Crisis', DPI/1485-94, backgrounder 1, press kit for World Summit for Social Development, United Nations, New York, July 1994
5. Brogan, Hugh, *The Pelican History of the United States*, Penguin Books/Viking, 1987, p. 107
6. Boutros-Ghali, Boutros, address to second session of the Preparatory Committee for the World Summit for Social Development, New York, 22 August 1994
7. Ibid.
8. Somavia, Juan, 'The Need for a New Ethic in International Relations', keynote address to International Press Service, Council on Information and Communication for International Development, Rome, 27 April 1993
9. The need to increase the efficiency of investment is a principal theme of the World Bank's *World Development Report 1994*
10. United Nations Children's Fund, *First Call for Children: World Declaration and Plan of Action from the World Summit for Children, and Convention on the Rights of the Child*, UNICEF, New York, December 1990
11. Editorial, *The New York Times*, 1 October 1990
12. World Health Organization, *Global Prevalence of Iodine Deficiency Disorders*, published jointly by WHO, UNICEF and the International Council for the Control of Iodine Deficiency Disorders, WHO, Geneva, 1993
13. *First Call for Children*, op. cit.
14. World Health Organization, 'Infant and Young Child Nutrition (Progress and Evaluation Report; and Status of Implementation of the International Code of Marketing of Breast-milk Substitutes)', A47/6, report by the Director-General, WHO, Geneva, March 1994, para. 164
15. Jonsson, Urban, 'Millions Lost to Wrong Strategies', in United Nations Children's Fund, *The Progress of Nations 1994*, UNICEF, New York, 1994, p. 7
16. United Nations Administrative Committee on Coordination, Subcommittee on Nutrition, *Controlling Vitamin A Deficiency*, Nutrition Policy Discussion Papers, No. 14, January 1994
17. World Health Organization, *The Prevalence of Anaemia in Women: A Tabulation of Available Information*, WHO, Geneva, 1992
18. World Health Organization, 'Infant and Young Child Nutrition', op. cit.
19. United Nations Children's Fund, World Health Organization, United Nations Educational, Scientific and Cultural Organization, and United Nations Population Fund, *Facts for Life: A Communications Challenge*, second edition, UNICEF, New York, 1993
20. World Health Organization and United Nations Children's Fund, 'Protecting, Promoting and Supporting Breastfeeding: The Special Role of Maternity Services', joint WHO/UNICEF statement, WHO, Geneva, 1989
21. Professor Yngve Hofvander, Department of Paediatrics, University Hospital, Uppsala, personal communication, 9 September 1994
22. World Health Organization, 'Infant and Young Child Nutrition', op. cit.
23. World Health Organization, Expanded Programme on Immunization, *Programme Report 1993*, WHO/EPI/GEN/94.1, WHO, Geneva, January 1994, p. 63
24. WHO and UNICEF data, reviewed in September 1994
25. World Health Organization, Global Programme for Vaccines, *Progress Towards the Global Eradication of Poliomyelitis: Status Report*, WHO/GPV/POLIO/94.1, WHO, Geneva, March 1994
26. Ibid.
27. World Health Organization, Expanded Programme on Immunization, *Programme Report 1993*, op. cit., p. 38
28. World Health Organization, Programme for Control of Diarrhoeal Diseases, *Programme Report 1993*, WHO/CDD/94.46, WHO, Geneva, 1994
29. World Health Organization, Programme for Control of Acute Respiratory Infections, *Interim Programme Report 1992*, WHO/ARI/93.25, WHO, Geneva, 1993
30. WHO Collaborating Center for Research, Training, and Eradication of Dracunculiasis at the US Centers for Disease Control, *Guinea Worm Wrap-up*, No. 42, January 1994
31. World Health Organization, 'Maternal and Child Health and Family Planning: Current Needs and Future Orientation', EB93/18, report by the Director-General, WHO, Geneva, 12 January 1993
32. Ibid., p. 5
33. Berstecher, D., and Carr-Hill, R., 'Primary Education and Economic Recession in the Developing World since 1980', study prepared for the World Conference on Education for All, Thailand, 5-9 March 1990, UNESCO, New York, 1990
34. Parker, David, and Jespersen, Eva, *20/20: Mobilizing Resources for Children in the 1990s*, UNICEF Staff Working Papers, No. 12, UNICEF, New York, 1994
35. World Health Organization, *The International Drinking Water Supply and Sanitation Decade: End of Decade Review*, WHO/CWS/92.12, WHO, Geneva, 1992
36. *First Call for Children*, op. cit.
37. Organisation for Economic Co-operation and Development, press release, SG/PRESS(94)46, Paris, 20 June 1994, p. 2
38. Organisation for Economic Co-operation and Development, cited in James Gustave Speth, UNDP Administrator, memorandum to UNICEF Executive Director, 29 June 1994
39. Cited in United Nations Children's Fund, *The State of the World's Children 1989*, UNICEF, New York, 1988, p. 9
40. Jolly, Richard 'The United Nations: A Development Agenda for the 21st Century', 1994 Ashby Lecture, Clare Hall, Cambridge, England, 10 March 1994

41 United Nations, 'Outcome of the World Summit for Social Development: Draft Declaration and Draft Programme of Action', A/CONF.166/PC/L.13, note by the Secretary-General to the Preparatory Committee for the World Summit for Social Development, United Nations, New York, 3 June 1994
42 Harrison, Paul, *The Third Revolution*, Penguin Books, London, 1992
43 'Philippines: The Answer's a Tomato', *The Economist*, 21 May 1994, p. 86
44 World Bank, *World Development Report 1994*, op. cit., table 30, p. 220
45 United Nations Development Programme, *Human Development Report 1994*, op. cit., p. 63
46 World Bank, *World Development Report 1994*, op. cit., p. 3
47 Overseas Development Council, 'Growth from Below: A People-oriented Development Strategy', Development Paper No. 16, ODC, Washington, D.C., December 1973
48 Galbraith, John Kenneth, 'The Challenge to the South: Seven Basic Principles', in *Facing the Challenge: Responses to the Report of the South Commission*, South Centre/Zed Books, London, 1993, p. 237
49 United Nations, op. cit., para. 41
50 United Nations Development Programme, United Nations Population Fund and United Nations Children's Fund, *The 20/20 Initiative: Achieving Universal Access to Basic Social Services for Sustainable Human Development*, UNDP, New York, 1994. The 20/20 theme is also discussed in recent editions of the UNDP *Human Development Report*
51 United Nations Development Programme, *Human Development Report 1994*, op. cit., p. 7
52 World Bank, *World Development Report 1993: Investing in Health*, World Bank, Washington, D.C., 1993
53 Rohde, Jon, Chatterjee, Meera, and Morley, David, eds., *Reaching Health for All*, Oxford University Press, 1993
54 World Bank, *World Development Report 1991*, World Bank, Washington, D.C., 1991, p. 66
55 United Nations Children's Fund and World Health Organization, 'Achieving the Mid-decade Goals for Water Supply and Sanitation', JCHPSS/94/2.11, UNICEF-WHO Joint Committee on Health Policy, special session, Geneva, 27-28 January 1994
56 World Bank, *World Development Report 1993*, op. cit.
57 Ibid.
58 Parker, David, and Jespersen, Eva, op. cit.
59 Organisation for Economic Co-operation and Development, press release, op. cit.
60 Kan, Shirley A., *Military Expenditures by Developing Countries: Foreign Aid Policy Issues*, report for Congress by Congressional Research Service, Library of Congress, Washington, D.C., 3 November 1993
61 Ibid.
62 United Nations Development Programme, *Human Development Report 1994*, op. cit.
63 United Nations Development Programme, United Nations Population Fund and United Nations Children's Fund, *The 20/20 Initiative*, op. cit., p. 8
64 World Bank, *World Development Report 1993*, op. cit.
65 This aspect is discussed in the *World Development Report 1994*
66 World Bank, *World Development Report 1993*, op. cit., p. 12
67 Ibid., p. 70
68 Wallerstein, Immanuel, 'Wise, but Not Tough, or is it Correct, but Not Wise?', in *Facing the Challenge: Responses to the Report of the South Commission*, South Centre/Zed Books, London, 1993, p. 117
69 Mosca, Gaetano, *The Ruling Class*, McGraw-Hill, New York, 1939, p. 50
70 Bruckner, Gene, *Renaissance Florence*, University of California Press, London, 1969, p. 139
71 Goubert, Pierre, *The French Peasantry in the Seventeenth Century*, Cambridge University Press, Cambridge, England, 1982, p. 197
72 Alexander, Cecil Frances, *All Things Bright and Beautiful*, second verse
73 da Costa, Emilia Viotti, in Bethell, Leslie, ed., *Brazil, Empire and Republic 1822-1930*, Cambridge University Press, Cambridge, England, 1989, p. 171
74 Kothari, Rajni, 'Towards a Politics of the South', in *Facing the Challenge: Responses to the Report of the South Commission*, South Centre/Zed Books, London, 1993, p. 84
75 World Bank, *World Development Report 1993*, op. cit., p. 23
76 Cited in United Nations, Department of Social Affairs, *Preliminary Report on the World Social Situation with Special Reference to Standards of Living*, United Nations, New York, 1952
77 Cited in Children's Defense Fund, *The State of America's Children 1994*, Children's Defense Fund, Washington, D.C., 1994
78 *The Economist*, 11 August 1994
79 Cited in Lasch, Christopher, *The True and Only Heaven: Progress and its Critics*, Norton Books, New York, 1991, p. 169
80 'In the bunker', *The Economist*, 8 January 1994, p. 63
81 Rothman, David J., 'The Crime of Punishment', *New York Review of Books*, 17 February 1994, p. 34
82 'The Future of Entertainment Networks', *PC Magazine* (UK edition), Vol. 3, No. 10, October 1994
83 'The Business of Wine', in Buckley, Richard, ed., *The World of Wine: The Grape and Civilisation, Understanding Global Issues*, European Schoolbooks Publishing, Cheltenham, England, 1994, p. 10
84 *The Economist Book of Vital World Statistics*, Economist Books/Hutchinson, London, 1990, pp. 239 and 243
85 Shaw, George Bernard, *Man and Superman*, Penguin Books/Viking, 1950

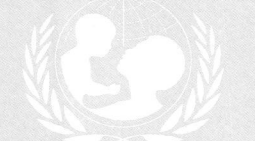

Statistical tables

Economic and social statistics on the nations of the world, with particular reference to children's well-being.

General note on the data	page 64	Country groupings	page 86
Explanation of symbols	page 64	Definitions	page 88
Index to countries	page 65	Main sources	page 89

Tables

1	Basic indicators	page 66	6	Economic indicators	page 76
2	Nutrition	page 68	7	Women	page 78
3	Health	page 70	8	Less populous countries	page 80
4	Education	page 72	9	The rate of progress	page 82
5	Demographic indicators	page 74	10	Regional summaries	page 84

GENERAL NOTE ON THE DATA

The data provided in these tables are accompanied by definitions, sources, and explanations of symbols. Tables derived from so many sources – 12 major sources are listed in the explanatory material – will inevitably cover a wide range of data reliability. Official government data received by the responsible United Nations agency have been used whenever possible. In the many cases where there are no reliable official figures, estimates made by the responsible United Nations agency have been used. Where such internationally standardized estimates do not exist, the tables draw on other sources, particularly data received from the appropriate UNICEF field office. Where possible only comprehensive or representative national data have been used.

Data for life expectancy, crude birth and death rates, infant mortality rates, etc., are part of the regular work on estimates and projections undertaken by the United Nations Population Division. These and other internationally produced estimates are revised periodically, which explains why some of the data will differ from those found in earlier UNICEF publications. Changes have been made to three indicators in this year's tables. The indicator in the education table for completion of primary school has been replaced with the percentage of school/grade 1 entrants reaching grade 5. In table 2 the wasting and stunting indicators now refer to all under-fives. These changes make the indicators consistent with those used in monitoring progress towards the World Summit for Children and mid-decade goals.

EXPLANATION OF SYMBOLS

Since the aim of the statistics section is to provide a broad picture of the situation of children and women worldwide, detailed data qualifications and footnotes are seen as more appropriate for inclusion elsewhere. Only two symbols are used in the tables.

.. Data not available

x Indicates data that refer to years or periods other than those specified in the column heading, differ from the standard definition, or refer to only part of a country.

Child mortality estimates for individual countries are primarily derived from data reported by the United Nations Population Division. In some cases, these estimates may differ from the latest national figures. In general, data released during approximately the last year are not incorporated in these estimates.

INDEX TO COUNTRIES

In the following tables, countries are ranked in descending order of their estimated 1993 under-five mortality rate. The reference numbers indicating that rank are given in the alphabetical list of countries below.

Country	Rank	Country	Rank	Country	Rank
Afghanistan	5	Georgia	93	Nigeria	18
Albania	79	Germany	138	Norway	137
Algeria	61	Ghana	25	Oman	92
Angola	2	Greece	123	Pakistan	33
Argentina	95	Guatemala	57	Panama	107
Armenia	86	Guinea	7	Papua New Guinea	49
Australia	131	Guinea-Bissau	6	Paraguay	85
Austria	135	Haiti	36	Peru	64
Azerbaijan	74	Honduras	72	Philippines	68
Bangladesh	39	Hong Kong*	140	Poland	115
Belarus	100	Hungary	116	Portugal	119
Belgium	124	India	40	Romania	91
Benin	30	Indonesia	45	Russian Federation	90
Bhutan	17	Iran, Islamic Rep. of	73	Rwanda	32
Bolivia	43	Iraq	59	Saudi Arabia	82
Botswana	71	Ireland	139	Senegal	42
Brazil	63	Israel	128	Sierra Leone	3
Bulgaria	108	Italy	129	Singapore	143
Burkina Faso	24	Jamaica	117	Slovakia	111
Burundi	22	Japan	142	Somalia	11
Cambodia	21	Jordan	94	South Africa	60
Cameroon	44	Kazakhstan	75	Spain	125
Canada	132	Kenya	50	Sri Lanka	109
Central African Rep.	23	Korea, Dem. Peo. Rep.	89	Sudan	37
Chad	12	Korea, Rep. of	127	Sweden	144
Chile	112	Kuwait	118	Switzerland	133
China	78	Kyrgyzstan	69	Syrian Arab Rep.	81
Colombia	110	Lao Peo. Dem. Rep.	31	Tajikistan	54
Congo	47	Latvia	96	Tanzania, U. Rep. of	26
Costa Rica	114	Lebanon	80	Thailand	87
Côte d'Ivoire	41	Lesotho	28	Togo	35
Cuba	120	Liberia	9	Trinidad and Tobago	104
Czech Rep.	122	Libyan Arab Jamahiriya	48	Tunisia	84
Denmark	141	Lithuania	106	Turkey	52
Dominican Rep.	76	Madagascar	27	Turkmenistan	51
Ecuador	70	Malawi	8	Uganda	20
Egypt	66	Malaysia	113	Ukraine	97
El Salvador	65	Mali	10	United Arab Emirates	103
Eritrea	13	Mauritania	16	United Kingdom	134
Estonia	99	Mauritius	101	United States	121
Ethiopia	14	Mexico	88	Uruguay	105
Finland	145	Moldova	83	Uzbekistan	62
France	126	Mongolia	56	Venezuela	98
Gabon	29	Morocco	67	Viet Nam	77
		Mozambique	4	Yemen	34
		Myanmar	46	Yugoslavia (former)	102
		Namibia	55	Zaire	19
		Nepal	38	Zambia	15
		Netherlands	136	Zimbabwe	53
		New Zealand	130		
		Nicaragua	58		
		Niger	1	*Colony.*	

Table 1: Basic indicators

		Under-5 mortality rate 1960	Under-5 mortality rate 1993	Infant mortality rate (under 1) 1960	Infant mortality rate (under 1) 1993	Total population (millions) 1993	Annual no. of births (thousands) 1993	Annual no. of under-5 deaths (thousands) 1993	GNP per capita (US$) 1992	Life expectancy at birth (years) 1993	Total adult literacy rate 1990	Primary school enrolment ratio (gross) 1986-1992	% share of household income 1980-1991 lowest 40%	% share of household income 1980-1991 highest 20%
1	Niger	320	**320**	191	191	8.5	439	140	280	47	28	29	..	..
2	Angola	345	**292**	208	170	10.3	529	154	610x	47	42	91	..	..
3	Sierra Leone	385	**284**	219	164	4.5	217	62	160	43	21	48	..	..
4	Mozambique	331	**282**	190	164	15.3	695	196	60	47	33	60	..	..
5	Afghanistan	360	**257**	215	165	20.6	1086	279	280x	44	29	24	..	..
6	Guinea-Bissau	336	**235**	200	139	1.0	44	10	220	44	37	60	9	59
7	Guinea	337	**226**	203	133	6.3	320	72	510	45	24	37	..	..
8	Malawi	365	**223**	206	141	10.7	580	130	210	44	49x	66	..	..
9	Liberia	288	**217**	192	145	2.9	135	29	450x	56	40	35	..	..
10	Mali	400	**217**	233	120	10.1	515	112	310	46	32	25	..	..
11	Somalia	294	**211**	175	125	9.5	480	101	150x	47	24	11x	..	..
12	Chad	325	**206**	195	121	6.0	264	54	220	48	30	65	..	..
13	Eritrea	294	**204**	175	120	3.4	146	30	110	48	..	..	..	..
14	Ethiopia	294	**204**	175	120	51.2	2681	547	110	47	24x	25	21	41
15	Zambia	220	**203**	135	114	8.9	411	83	290	44	73	92	15	50
16	Mauritania	321	**202**	191	116	2.2	102	21	530	48	34	55	14	46
17	Bhutan	324	**197**	203	128	1.7	66	13	180	49	38	25	..	..
18	Nigeria	204	**191**	122	114	119.3	5353	1022	320	53	51	71	..	..
19	Zaire	286	**187**	167	120	41.2	1959	366	230x	52	72	76	..	..
20	Uganda	218	**185**	129	111	19.3	983	182	170	42	48	80	21	42
21	Cambodia	217	**181**	146	115	9.0	351	63	200x	51	35	..	..	..
22	Burundi	255	**178**	151	107	6.0	276	49	210	48	50	70	..	..
23	Central African Rep.	294	**177**	174	104	3.3	145	26	410	47	38	68	..	..
24	Burkina Faso	318	**175**	183	99	9.8	458	80	300	48	18	37	..	..
25	Ghana	215	**170**	128	103	16.5	683	116	450	56	60	77	18	44
26	Tanzania, U. Rep. of	249	**167**	147	108	28.8	1387	232	110	51	46x	69	8	63
27	Madagascar	364	**164**	219	100	13.3	604	99	230	56	80	92	..	..
28	Lesotho	204	**156**	138	107	1.9	65	10	590	61	..	107	9	60
29	Gabon	287	**154**	171	93	1.3	55	8	4450	54	61	..	..	..
30	Benin	310	**144**	184	87	5.1	249	36	410	46	23	66	..	..
31	Lao Peo. Dem. Rep.	233	**141**	155	96	4.6	209	29	250	51	84x	98	..	..
32	Rwanda	191	**141**	115	81	7.8	407	57	250	46	50	71	23	39
33	Pakistan	221	**137**	137	95	128.1	5162	707	420	59	35	42	21	40
34	Yemen	378	**137**	214	91	13.0	623	85	520	53	39	78	..	..
35	Togo	264	**135**	155	84	3.9	173	23	390	55	43	111	..	..
36	Haiti	270	**130**	182	85	6.9	243	32	370	57	53	56	..	..
37	Sudan	292	**128**	170	77	27.4	1146	147	420x	52	27	50	..	..
38	Nepal	279	**128**	186	90	21.1	782	100	170	54	26	82	22	40
39	Bangladesh	247	**122**	151	94	122.2	4712	575	220	53	35	77	23	39
40	India	236	**122**	144	81	896.6	26063	3167	310	61	48	98	21	41
41	Côte d'Ivoire	300	**120**	165	89	13.4	670	81	670	51	54	69	19	42
42	Senegal	303	**120**	174	63	8.0	340	41	780	49	38	59	11	59
43	Bolivia	252	**114**	152	78	7.7	264	30	680	61	77	85	15	48
44	Cameroon	264	**113**	156	71	12.6	510	58	820	56	54	101	..	..
45	Indonesia	216	**111**	127	71	194.6	5149	572	670	63	82	116	21	42
46	Myanmar	237	**111**	158	81	44.6	1446	160	220x	58	81	97	..	..
47	Congo	220	**109**	143	82	2.4	109	12	1030	51	57	..	..	..
48	Libyan Arab Jamahiriya	269	**100**	160	67	5.1	211	21	5310x	63	64	..	..	..
49	Papua New Guinea	248	**95**	165	67	4.2	139	13	950	56	52	71	..	..
50	Kenya	202	**90**	120	61	26.1	1139	103	310	59	69	95	10	62
51	Turkmenistan	..	**89**	..	71	4.0	131	12	1230	66	98x	..	..	..
52	Turkey	217	**84**	161	67	59.6	1663	139	1980	67	81	113	..	..
53	Zimbabwe	181	**83**	109	58	10.9	441	37	570	56	67	119	10	62
54	Tajikistan	..	**83**	..	64	5.8	222	18	490	69	98x	..	..	..
55	Namibia	206	**79**	129	62	1.6	68	5	1610	59	..	119	..	..
56	Mongolia	185	**78**	128	59	2.4	80	6	780x	64	..	89	..	..
57	Guatemala	205	**73**	137	53	10.0	387	28	980	65	55	79	8	63
58	Nicaragua	209	**72**	140	51	4.1	165	12	340	67	35x	101	..	..
59	Iraq	171	**71**	117	57	19.9	770	55	1500x	66	60	111	..	..
60	South Africa	126	**69**	89	53	40.8	1270	88	2670	63	..	76x	..	..
61	Algeria	243	**68**	148	57	27.1	920	63	1840	66	57	95	18	47
62	Uzbekistan	..	**66**	..	54	22.0	704	46	850	69	97x	..	..	..
63	Brazil	181	**63**	118	52	156.6	3590	226	2770	66	82	106	7	68
64	Peru	236	**62**	143	43	22.9	662	41	950	65	85	126	14	51
65	El Salvador	210	**60**	130	45	5.5	185	11	1170	67	73	76	..	..
66	Egypt	258	**59**	169	46	56.1	1733	102	640	62	48	101	..	..
67	Morocco	215	**59**	133	48	27.0	861	50	1030	64	50	66	17	46
68	Philippines	102	**59**	73	45	66.5	1999	117	770	65	94	110	17	48
69	Kyrgyzstan	..	**58**	..	48	4.6	128	7	820	66	96x	..	..	..
70	Ecuador	180	**57**	115	45	11.3	333	19	1070	67	87	116	..	..
71	Botswana	170	**56**	117	43	1.4	52	3	2790	61	74	119	11	59
72	Honduras	203	**56**	137	43	5.6	207	12	580	66	73	105	9	64
73	Iran, Islamic Rep. of	233	**54**	145	42	63.2	2507	136	2200	67	54	112	..	..
74	Azerbaijan	..	**52**	..	36	7.4	163	8	740	71	97x	..	..	..
75	Kazakhstan	..	**49**	..	42	17.1	308	15	1680	69	97x	..	..	..

		Under-5 mortality rate		Infant mortality rate (under 1)		Total population (millions) 1993	Annual no. of births (thousands) 1993	Annual no. of under-5 deaths (thousands) 1993	GNP per capita (US$) 1992	Life expectancy at birth (years) 1993	Total adult literacy rate 1990	Primary school enrolment ratio (gross) 1986-1992	% share of household income 1980-1991	
		1960	1993	1960	1993								lowest 40%	highest 20%
76	Dominican Rep.	152	**48**	104	40	7.6	213	10	1050	68	83	95	12	56
77	Viet Nam	219	**48**	147	36	70.9	2055	98	240x	64	88	103	..	..
78	China	209	**43**	140	35	1205.2	24903	1071	470	71	78	123	17	42
79	Albania	151	**41**	112	34	3.3	75	3	790x	73	..	101	..	..
80	Lebanon	85	**40**	65	33	2.9	79	3	2150x	69	80	112	..	..
81	Syrian Arab Rep.	201	**39**	136	33	13.8	583	23	1160	67	64	109	..	..
82	Saudi Arabia	292	**38**	170	33	16.5	590	22	7510	69	62	77	..	..
83	Moldova	..	**36**	..	31	4.4	65	2	1300	68	96x	..	..	..
84	Tunisia	244	**36**	163	30	8.6	231	8	1720	68	65	117	16	46
85	Paraguay	90	**34**	66	28	4.6	153	5	1380	67	90	109	..	..
86	Armenia	..	**33**	..	28	3.5	71	2	780	72	99x	..	..	..
87	Thailand	146	**33**	101	27	56.9	1157	38	1840	69	93	90	16	51
88	Mexico	141	**32**	98	27	90.0	2499	81	3470	70	88	114	12	56
89	Korea, Dem. Peo. Rep.	120	**32**	85	24	23.1	559	18	970x	71	..	104	..	..
90	Russian Federation	..	**31**	..	28	148.3	1779	55	2510	69	99x	..	..	..
91	Romania	82	**29**	69	23	23.4	365	11	1130	70	97	90	..	..
92	Oman	300	**29**	180	23	1.7	68	2	6480	70	..	100	..	..
93	Georgia	..	**28**	..	24	5.5	83	2	850	73	99x	..	..	..
94	Jordan	149	**27**	103	23	4.4	176	5	1120	68	80	97	17	48
95	Argentina	68	**27**	57	24	33.5	676	18	6050	71	95	107	..	..
96	Latvia	..	**26**	..	22	2.7	36	1	1930	71	99x	..	..	..
97	Ukraine	..	**25**	..	21	51.9	622	16	1820	70	98x	..	..	..
98	Venezuela	70	**24**	53	20	20.6	533	13	2910	70	88	99	14	50
99	Estonia	..	**23**	..	20	1.6	22	1	2760	72	100x	..	..	..
100	Belarus	..	**22**	..	19	10.4	135	3	2930	71	98x	..	..	..
101	Mauritius	84	**22**	62	19	1.1	20	0	2700	70	80	106	..	..
102	Yugoslavia (former)	113	**22**	92	19	24.0	337	7	3060x	72	93	94	..	..
103	United Arab Emirates	240	**21**	160	18	1.7	36	1	22020	71	53x	115	..	..
104	Trinidad and Tobago	73	**21**	61	18	1.3	30	1	3940	71	95x	96	..	..
105	Uruguay	47	**21**	41	19	3.2	54	1	3340	72	96	110	..	..
106	Lithuania	..	**20**	..	17	3.8	55	1	1310	73	98x	..	8	60
107	Panama	104	**20**	67	18	2.6	64	1	2420	73	89	106	..	..
108	Bulgaria	70	**19**	49	16	8.9	111	2	1330	72	..	92	24	36
109	Sri Lanka	130	**19**	90	15	17.9	370	7	540	72	88	108	22	39
110	Colombia	132	**19**	82	16	34.0	809	15	1330	69	87	111	11	56
111	Slovakia	..	**18**	..	16	5.4	81	1	1930	72	..	..	11	63
112	Chile	138	**17**	107	15	13.8	309	5	2730	72	93	98	13	54
113	Malaysia	105	**17**	73	13	19.2	543	9	2790	71	78	93	13	51
114	Costa Rica	112	**16**	80	14	3.3	85	1	1960	76	93	103	23	36
115	Poland	70	**15**	62	13	38.5	547	8	1910	72	99x	98	26	34
116	Hungary	57	**15**	51	13	10.5	129	2	2970	70	99x	89	16	48
117	Jamaica	76	**13**	58	11	2.5	55	1	1340	74	98	106	..	..
118	Kuwait	128	**13**	89	11	1.8	53	1	16150x	75	73	55	..	..
119	Portugal	112	**11**	81	9	9.9	114	1	7450	75	85	122	..	..
120	Cuba	50	**10**	39	9	10.9	190	2	1170x	76	94	102	..	..
121	United States	30	**10**	26	9	257.8	4093	42	23240	76	..	104	16	42
122	Czech Rep.	..	**10**	..	9	10.4	146	1	2450	72	..	..	..	..
123	Greece	64	**10**	53	9	10.2	106	1	7290	78	93	97	..	..
124	Belgium	35	**10**	31	8	10.0	122	1	20880	76	..	99	22x	36x
125	Spain	57	**9**	46	8	39.2	426	4	13970	78	95	109	22	37
126	France	34	**9**	29	7	57.4	772	7	22260	77	..	107	17	42
127	Korea, Rep. of	124	**9**	88	8	44.5	731	7	6790	71	96	105	20	42
128	Israel	39	**9**	32	7	5.4	112	1	13220	77	92x	95	18x	40x
129	Italy	50	**9**	44	7	57.8	583	5	20460	77	97	94	19	41
130	New Zealand	26	**9**	22	7	3.5	61	1	12300	76	..	104	16	45
131	Australia	24	**8**	20	7	17.8	269	2	17260	77	..	107	16	42
132	Canada	33	**8**	28	7	27.8	394	3	20710	77	97x	107	18	40
133	Switzerland	27	**8**	22	6	6.9	87	1	36080	78	..	103	17	45
134	United Kingdom	27	**8**	23	7	57.8	803	6	17790	76	..	104	15	44
135	Austria	43	**8**	37	7	7.8	91	1	22380	76	..	103	..	..
136	Netherlands	22	**8**	18	6	15.3	212	2	20480	77	..	102	21	37
137	Norway	23	**8**	19	6	4.3	64	0	25820	77	..	100	19x	37x
138	Germany	40	**7**	34	6	80.6	917	7	23030	76	..	105	19	40
139	Ireland	36	**7**	31	6	3.5	50	0	12210	75	..	103	..	..
140	Hong Kong	52	**7**	38	6	5.9	75	1	15360	78	77x	108	16	47
141	Denmark	25	**7**	22	6	5.2	65	0	26000	76	..	96	17	39
142	Japan	40	**6**	31	5	125.0	1407	9	28190	79	..	102	22x	38x
143	Singapore	40	**6**	31	5	2.8	44	0	15730	75	83x	108	15	49
144	Sweden	20	**6**	16	5	8.7	122	1	27010	78	..	100	21	37
145	Finland	28	**5**	22	4	5.0	65	0	21970	76	..	99	18	38

Countries listed in descending order of their under-five mortality rates (shown in bold type).

Table 2: Nutrition

		% of infants with low birth weight 1990	% of children (1986-93) who are: exclusively breastfed (0-3 months)	breastfed with complementary food (6-9 months)	still breastfeeding (20-23 months)	% of under-fives (1980-93) suffering from: underweight moderate & severe	underweight severe	wasting moderate & severe	stunting moderate & severe	Total goitre rate (6-11 years) (%) 1980-92	Daily per capita calorie supply as a % of requirements 1988-90	% share of total household consumption (1980-85) all food	cereals
1	Niger	15	..	..	..	36	12	16	32	9	95	..	..
2	Angola	19	3	83	53	..	..	..	..	7	80	..	..
3	Sierra Leone	17	..	94	41	29	..	9x	35	7	83	56	22
4	Mozambique	20	..	..	..	..	..	..	..	20	77	..	..
5	Afghanistan	20	..	..	..	..	..	..	..	20	72	..	..
6	Guinea-Bissau	20	..	..	..	23x	..	..	..	19	97	..	..
7	Guinea	21	..	..	..	..	..	..	..	19	97	..	..
8	Malawi	20	3	89	..	27	8	5	49	13	88	30	9
9	Liberia	..	15	56	26	20x	..	3x	37x	6	98	..	..
10	Mali	17	8	45	44	31x	9x	11x	24x	29	96	57	22
11	Somalia	16	..	..	..	..	..	..	..	7	81	..	..
12	Chad	..	..	..	..	..	..	..	..	15	73	..	..
13	Eritrea	..	..	..	..	..	..	..	..	..	..	..	..
14	Ethiopia	16	74	..	35	48x	16x	8x	64x	22	73	49	24
15	Zambia	13	13	88	34	25	6	5	40	51x	87	36	8
16	Mauritania	11	12	39	..	48	..	16	57	..	106	..	..
17	Bhutan	..	..	..	..	38	..	4	56	25	128	..	..
18	Nigeria	16	2	52	43	36	12	9	43	10	93	48	18
19	Zaire	15	..	..	..	28x	..	5x	43x	9	96	..	..
20	Uganda	..	70	67	39	23	5	2	45	7	93	..	..
21	Cambodia	..	..	..	..	..	..	..	..	15	96	..	..
22	Burundi	..	89	66	73	38x	10x	6x	48x	42	84	..	..
23	Central African Rep.	15	..	..	..	..	..	..	..	63	82	..	..
24	Burkina Faso	21x	3	35	..	30	8	13	29	16	94	..	..
25	Ghana	17	2	57	52	27	6	7	31	10	93	50	..
26	Tanzania, U. Rep. of	14	32	89	57	29	7	6	47	37	95	64	32
27	Madagascar	10	47	93	45	39	9	5	51	24	95	59	26
28	Lesotho	11	..	..	..	16	2	5	26	16	93	..	..
29	Gabon	..	..	..	..	..	..	..	..	5	104	..	..
30	Benin	..	..	..	..	..	..	..	..	24	104	37	12
31	Lao Peo. Dem. Rep.	18	..	..	..	37	..	11	40	25	111	..	..
32	Rwanda	17	90	75	..	29	6	4	48	49	82	29	10
33	Pakistan	25	25	29	52	40	14	9	50	32	99	37	12
34	Yemen	19	15	51	..	30	4	13	44	32	..	..	..
35	Togo	20	10	86	68	24x	6x	5x	30x	22	99	..	..
36	Haiti	15	..	..	..	37x	3x	9x	40x	4	89	..	..
37	Sudan	15	14	45	44	20	..	14	32	20	87	60	..
38	Nepal	..	..	..	..	70x	5x	14x	69x	44	100	57	38
39	Bangladesh	50	..	..	..	66x	27x	16x	65x	11	88	59	36
40	India	33	..	..	..	69x	27x	..	65x	9	101	52	18
41	Côte d'Ivoire	14x	..	..	..	12	2	9	17	6	111	39	13
42	Senegal	11	9	42	95	20	5	9	22	12	98	49	15
43	Bolivia	12	59	57	30	13x	3x	2x	38x	21	84	33	..
44	Cameroon	13	7	77	35	14	3	3	24	26	95	24	7
45	Indonesia	14	53	76	62	40	..	..	..	28	121	48	21
46	Myanmar	16	..	..	..	32x	9x	..	..	18	114	..	..
47	Congo	16	43	..	27	24	..	5	27	8	103	37	16
48	Libyan Arab Jamahiriya	..	..	..	..	..	..	..	..	6	140	..	..
49	Papua New Guinea	23	..	..	..	35	..	..	..	30	114	..	..
50	Kenya	16	17	97	54	22	6	6	33	7	89	38	16
51	Turkmenistan	..	..	..	..	..	..	..	..	20	..	..	..
52	Turkey	8	..	..	..	..	..	..	..	36	127	40	9
53	Zimbabwe	14	11	94	26	12x	2x	1x	29x	42	94	40	9
54	Tajikistan	..	..	..	..	..	..	..	..	20	..	..	..
55	Namibia	12	22	65	23	26	6	9	28	35	..	..	..
56	Mongolia	10	..	..	..	12x	..	2x	26x	7	97	..	..
57	Guatemala	14	..	..	44	34x	8x	1x	58x	20	103	36	10
58	Nicaragua	15	..	..	..	11	1	1	22	4	99	..	..
59	Iraq	15	..	..	..	12	2	3	22	7	128	..	..
60	South Africa	..	..	..	..	..	..	..	..	2	128	34	..
61	Algeria	9	..	..	..	9	..	6	18	9	123	..	..
62	Uzbekistan	..	..	..	..	..	..	..	..	18	..	..	..
63	Brazil	11	4	27	13	7	1	2	16	14x	114	35	9
64	Peru	11	40	62	36	11	2	1	37	36	87	35	8
65	El Salvador	11	..	..	..	15	..	5	30	25	102	33	12
66	Egypt	10	38	52	..	9	2	3	24	5	132	49	10
67	Morocco	9	48	48	18	9	2	2	23	20	125	38	12
68	Philippines	15	33	61	18	34	5	6	37	15	104	51	21
69	Kyrgyzstan	..	..	..	..	..	..	..	..	20	..	..	..
70	Ecuador	11	31	31	23	17	0	2	34	10	105	30	..
71	Botswana	8	41	82	23	15x	..	..	44	8	97	25	12
72	Honduras	9	..	..	..	21	4	2	34	9	98	39	..
73	Iran, Islamic Rep. of	9	..	..	..	..	..	..	..	30	125	37	10
74	Azerbaijan	..	..	..	..	..	..	..	..	20	..	..	..
75	Kazakhstan	..	..	..	..	..	..	..	..	20	..	..	..

		% of infants with low birth weight 1990	% of children (1986-93) who are: exclusively breastfed (0-3 months)	breastfed with complementary food (6-9 months)	still breastfeeding (20-23 months)	% of under-fives (1980-93) suffering from: underweight moderate & severe	severe	wasting moderate & severe	stunting moderate & severe	Total goitre rate (6-11 years) (%) 1980-92	Daily per capita calorie supply as a % of requirements 1988-90	% share of total household consumption (1980-85) all food	cereals
76	Dominican Rep.	16	10	23	7	10	2	1	19	..	102	46	13
77	Viet Nam	17	..	..	..	52	14	7	60	20	103	..	..
78	China	9	..	..	..	21x	3x	4x	32x	9	112	61	..
79	Albania	7	..	..	..	..	..	..	..	41	107	..	..
80	Lebanon	10	..	..	..	..	..	..	..	15	127	..	..
81	Syrian Arab Rep.	11	..	..	..	..	..	..	..	73	126	..	..
82	Saudi Arabia	7	..	..	..	..	..	..	..	..	121	..	..
83	Moldova	..	..	..	..	..	..	..	..	..	..	..	..
84	Tunisia	8	21	53	25	10x	2x	3x	18x	4	131	37	7
85	Paraguay	8	7	61	8	4	1	0	17	49	116	30	6
86	Armenia	..	..	..	..	..	..	..	..	10	..	..	..
87	Thailand	13	4	69	34	26x	4x	6x	22x	12	103	30	7
88	Mexico	12	37	36	21	14	..	6	22	15	131	35	..
89	Korea, Dem. Peo. Rep.	..	..	..	..	..	..	..	..	..	121	..	..
90	Russian Federation	..	..	..	..	..	..	..	..	..	..	..	..
91	Romania	7	..	..	..	..	..	..	..	10	116	..	..
92	Oman	10	..	..	..	..	..	..	..	..	..	..	..
93	Georgia	..	..	..	..	..	..	..	..	20	..	..	..
94	Jordan	7	32	48	13	6	1	3	19	..	110	35	..
95	Argentina	8	..	..	..	..	..	..	..	8	131	35	4
96	Latvia	..	..	..	..	..	..	..	..	..	..	..	..
97	Ukraine	..	..	..	..	..	..	..	..	10	..	..	..
98	Venezuela	9	..	..	..	6	..	2	6	11	99	23	..
99	Estonia	..	..	..	..	..	..	..	..	..	..	..	..
100	Belarus	..	..	..	..	..	..	..	..	22	..	..	..
101	Mauritius	9	..	..	..	24	..	16	22	..	128	24	7
102	Yugoslavia (former)	..	..	..	..	..	..	..	..	5	140	27	4
103	United Arab Emirates	6	..	..	26	..	..	..	..	..	..	..	..
104	Trinidad and Tobago	10	10	39	16	7x	0x	4x	5x	..	114	19	3
105	Uruguay	8	..	..	..	7	2	..	16	..	101	31	7
106	Lithuania	..	..	..	..	..	..	..	..	..	..	..	..
107	Panama	10	..	..	..	16	..	6	22	13	98	38	7
108	Bulgaria	6	..	..	..	..	..	..	..	20	148	..	..
109	Sri Lanka	25	14	47	46	29x	2x	18	36	14	101	43	18
110	Colombia	10	17	48	24	10	2	3	17	10	106	29	..
111	Slovakia	..	..	..	..	..	..	..	..	..	..	..	..
112	Chile	7	..	..	..	3x	..	1x	10x	9	102	29	7
113	Malaysia	10	..	..	..	..	..	..	..	20	120	23	..
114	Costa Rica	6	..	..	..	6	..	2	8	3	121	33	8
115	Poland	..	..	..	..	..	..	..	..	10	131	29	4
116	Hungary	9	..	..	..	..	..	..	..	..	137	25	3
117	Jamaica	11	..	..	..	7	1	3	9	..	114	36	14
118	Kuwait	7	..	..	..	6	..	3	12	..	..	..	..
119	Portugal	5	..	..	..	..	..	..	..	15	136	34	8
120	Cuba	8	..	..	..	..	..	1	..	10	135	..	..
121	United States	7	..	..	..	..	..	..	..	..	138	10	2
122	Czech Rep.	..	..	..	..	..	..	..	..	10	151	30	3
123	Greece	6	..	..	..	..	..	..	..	5	149	15	2
124	Belgium	6	..	..	..	..	..	..	..	10	141	24	3
125	Spain	4	..	..	..	..	..	..	..	5	143	16	3
126	France	5	..	..	..	..	..	..	..	..	120	35	14
127	Korea, Rep. of	9	..	..	..	..	..	..	..	..	125	21	..
128	Israel	7	..	..	..	..	..	..	..	20	139	19	2
129	Italy	5	..	..	..	..	..	..	..	..	131	12	2
130	New Zealand	6	..	..	..	..	..	..	..	..	131	12	2
131	Australia	6	..	..	..	..	..	..	..	..	124	13	2
132	Canada	6	..	..	..	..	..	..	..	..	122	11	2
133	Switzerland	5	..	..	..	..	..	..	..	..	130	17	..
134	United Kingdom	7	..	..	..	..	..	..	..	..	130	12	2
135	Austria	6	..	..	..	..	..	..	..	..	133	16	2
136	Netherlands	..	..	..	..	..	..	..	..	3	114	13	2
137	Norway	4	..	..	..	..	..	..	..	..	120	15	2
138	Germany	..	..	..	..	..	..	..	..	10	..	12	2
139	Ireland	4	..	..	..	..	..	..	..	..	157	22	4
140	Hong Kong	8	..	..	..	..	..	..	..	..	125	12	1
141	Denmark	6	..	..	..	..	..	..	..	5	135	13	2
142	Japan	6	..	..	..	..	..	..	..	..	125	17	4
143	Singapore	7	..	..	..	14x	..	4x	11x	..	136	19	..
144	Sweden	5	..	..	..	..	..	..	..	..	111	13	2
145	Finland	4	..	..	..	..	..	..	..	..	113	16	3

Countries listed in descending order of their 1993 under-five mortality rates (table 1).

Table 3: Health

		% of population with access to safe water 1988-93			% of population with access to adequate sanitation 1988-93			% of population with access to health services 1985-93			% fully immunized 1990-93					pregnant women tetanus	ORT use rate 1987-93
											1-year-old children					
		total	urban	rural	total	urban	rural	total	urban	rural	TB	DPT	polio	measles		
1	Niger	59	60	59	14	71	4	32	99	30	34	20	20	20	43	17
2	Angola	41	71	20	19	25	15	30x	..	..	53	30	28	47	14	48
3	Sierra Leone	37	33	37	58	92	49	38	90	20	79	63	63	67	81	60
4	Mozambique	22	44	17	20	61	11	39	100	30	66	49	49	62	24	60
5	Afghanistan	23	40	19	..	13	..	29	80	17	60	34	34	42	9	26
6	Guinea-Bissau	41	56	35	31	27	32	40	..	..	92	45	45	46	62	26
7	Guinea	55	50	56	21	84	10	80	100	70	76	55	55	57	61	82
8	Malawi	56x	97x	50x	60	30	81	80	..	..	96	92	92	92	69	50
9	Liberia	50	93	22	..	..	8	39	50	30	86	20	39	38	20	15
10	Mali	41	53	38	24	81	10	..	..	..	77	46	46	51	45	10
11	Somalia	37	50	29	18	44	5	27x	50x	15x	31x	18x	18x	30x	5x	78
12	Chad	..	30	..	..	..	..	30	64	..	34	13	13	19	4	15
13	Eritrea	..	..	..	..	..	..	..	..	..	37	28	28	23	4	..
14	Ethiopia	25	91	19	19	97	7	46	..	..	46	28	28	22	12	68
15	Zambia	53	70	28	37	75	12	75x	100x	50x	88	64	62	62	18	90
16	Mauritania	66	67	65	..	34	..	45	72	33	84	44	44	49	36	54
17	Bhutan	34	60	30	13	50	7	65	..	..	93	84	85	68	43	85
18	Nigeria	36	81	30	35	40	30	66	85	62	43	29	29	34	33	35
19	Zaire	39	68	24	23	46	11	26	40	17	43	29	29	33	25	46
20	Uganda	31	58	28	57	94	52	49x	99x	42x	99	73	74	73	83	45
21	Cambodia	36	65	33	14	81	8	53	80	50	57	35	36	37	22	6
22	Burundi	57	99	54	49	71	47	80	100	79	75	63	64	61	56	49
23	Central African Rep.	24	19	26	46	45	46	45	..	..	90	60	60	69	43	24
24	Burkina Faso	56	51	72	25	88	15	49x	51x	48x	72	47	47	42	36	15
25	Ghana	52	93	35	42	64	32	60	92	45	70	48	47	50	6	44
26	Tanzania, U. Rep. of	50	67	46	64	74	62	76x	99x	72x	92	82	81	79	15	76
27	Madagascar	23	55	9	3	12	3	65	65	65	82	64	64	52	16	29
28	Lesotho	47	59	45	22	14	23	80	..	..	98	80	76	77	34	78
29	Gabon	68	90	50	..	..	..	90x	..	..	97	66	66	65	86	25
30	Benin	51	66	46	34	42	31	18	..	..	88	75	72	67	77	28
31	Lao Peo. Dem. Rep.	36	54	33	21	97	8	67	..	..	42	25	26	46	24	55
32	Rwanda	66	75	62	58	77	56	80	..	..	94	85	85	81	88	47
33	Pakistan	68	85	50	38	60	17	55	99	35	87	74	74	71	46	59
34	Yemen	36	61	30	65	87	60	38	81	32	77	54	54	51	12	30
35	Togo	60	77	53	23	56	10	61	..	..	75	53	53	48	81	33
36	Haiti	39	55	33	24	55	16	50	..	..	48	30	30	24	12	20
37	Sudan	48	55	43	75	89	65	51	90	40	61	51	51	49	9	47
38	Nepal	42	67	39	6	52	3	..	..	..	73	64	64	59	13	49
39	Bangladesh	84	82	85	31	63	26	45	..	..	95	74	74	71	80	26
40	India	79	85	78	27	62	12	85	100	80	92	90	90	82	77	37
41	Côte d'Ivoire	76	70	81	60	59	62	30x	61x	11x	53	50	50	52	51	15
42	Senegal	48	84	26	55	85	36	40	..	..	69	52	52	46	30	18
43	Bolivia	54	81	19	43	63	17	67	77	52	84	81	83	81	52	63
44	Cameroon	50	57	43	74	100	64	41	44	39	41	33	33	33	49	84
45	Indonesia	51	68	43	44	64	36	80	..	..	94	89	93	90	67	78
46	Myanmar	32	37	..	36	39	35	48	..	..	80	73	73	71	66	37
47	Congo	38	92	2	..	..	..	83	97	70	63	60	60	55	53	67
48	Libyan Arab Jamahiriya	97	100	80	98	100	85	..	..	..	91	91	91	89	45	80
49	Papua New Guinea	33	94	20	20	57	10	96	..	..	65	37	35	30	27	51
50	Kenya	49	74	43	43	69	35	77	..	40	95	85	85	76	72	76
51	Turkmenistan	..	..	..	..	..	..	..	..	..	98	99	99	98	..	..
52	Turkey	78x	95x	63x	..	..	..	..	..	..	63	79	79	74	22	57
53	Zimbabwe	84	95	80	40	95	22	85	96	80	79	69	69	73	60	82
54	Tajikistan	..	..	..	..	..	..	..	..	..	69	82	74	97	..	..
55	Namibia	52	98	35	14	24	11	72	92	60	92	73	79	71	40	75
56	Mongolia	80	100	58	74	100	47	95	..	..	84	80	79	84	..	65
57	Guatemala	62	92	43	60	72	52	34	47	25	46	75	77	71	18	24
58	Nicaragua	54	76	21	..	78	18	83	100	60	94	78	94	83	12	40
59	Iraq	77	93	41	..	96	..	93	97	78	79	82	82	81	44	70
60	South Africa	..	..	..	..	..	..	..	..	..	66	79	79	85	26	..
61	Algeria	68x	85x	55x	79	96	60	88	100	80	87	73	73	69	36	27
62	Uzbekistan	..	..	..	..	..	..	..	..	..	89	58	51	91	..	..
63	Brazil	87	95	61	72	84	32	..	..	..	98	75	66	84	21	63
64	Peru	72	75	18	57	58	25	75x	..	..	87	84	86	75	30	31
65	El Salvador	47	85	19	58	86	36	40	80	40	79	79	79	86	26	45
66	Egypt	90	95	86	50	80	26	99	100	99	95	89	89	89	78	34
67	Morocco	54	92	14	65	95	38	70	100	50	91	86	86	83	80	17
68	Philippines	82	85	79	69	79	62	76	77	74	90	88	89	87	66	63
69	Kyrgyzstan	..	..	..	..	..	..	..	..	..	96	88	91	94	..	..
70	Ecuador	55	63	43	48	56	38	88	70	20	99	76	79	73	5	70
71	Botswana	89	100	77	55	91	41	89x	100x	85x	50	57	57	60	46	64
72	Honduras	68	89	51	63	90	57	66	80	56	95	94	95	94	16	70
73	Iran, Islamic Rep. of	89	100	75	71	100	35	80	95	65	99	99	99	96	50	85
74	Azerbaijan	..	..	..	..	..	..	..	..	..	94	71	70	84	..	..
75	Kazakhstan	..	..	..	..	..	..	..	..	..	93	76	69	91	..	..

		% of population with access to safe water 1988-93			% of population with access to adequate sanitation 1988-93			% of population with access to health services 1985-93			% fully immunized 1990-93				pregnant women tetanus	ORT use rate 1987-93
											1-year-old children				
		total	urban	rural	total	urban	rural	total	urban	rural	TB	DPT	polio	measles		
76	Dominican Rep.	59	75	35	87	95	75	80	..	..	84	57	82	99	24	37
77	Viet Nam	24	39	21	17	34	13	90	100	80	94	91	91	93	71	52
78	China	69	99	60	16	58	3	90	100	88	93	95	95	94	3	22
79	Albania	..	..	..	..	..	..	..	..	..	82	96	98	76	..	..
80	Lebanon	92	95	85	75x	94x	18x	95	98	85	4	87	87	65	..	45
81	Syrian Arab Rep.	74	90	58	83	84	82	90	96	84	91	90	90	86	86	95
82	Saudi Arabia	95	100	74	86	100	30	97	100	88	94	93	94	92	63	90
83	Moldova	..	..	..	..	..	..	..	..	..	96	87	97	92	..	..
84	Tunisia	99	100	99	96	98	94	90x	100x	80x	81	98	98	89	50	22
85	Paraguay	35	50	24	62	56	67	63	90	38	95	79	80	96	54	52
86	Armenia	..	..	..	..	..	..	..	..	..	88	85	92	93	..	..
87	Thailand	77	87	72	74	80	72	90	90	90	98	92	92	86	86	65
88	Mexico	84	94	66	50	70	17	78	80	60	97	94	95	93	68	81
89	Korea, Dem. Peo. Rep.	..	..	..	..	..	..	..	..	..	99	90	99	99	97	85
90	Russian Federation	..	..	..	..	..	..	..	..	..	86	62	69	83	..	..
91	Romania	..	..	..	..	..	..	..	..	..	99	98	92	91	..	..
92	Oman	84	91	77	71	75	40	96	100	94	95	97	97	95	95	72
93	Georgia	..	..	..	..	..	..	..	..	..	63	45	45	58	..	..
94	Jordan	99	100	97	100	100	100	97	98	95	..	95	95	88	30	53
95	Argentina	71	77	29	68	73	37	71	80	21	96	79	80	95	..	80
96	Latvia	..	..	..	..	..	..	..	..	..	91	79	83	80	..	..
97	Ukraine	..	..	..	..	..	..	..	..	..	93	88	89	90	..	..
98	Venezuela	89	89	89	92	97	70	..	..	..	82	69	75	63	60	80
99	Estonia	..	..	..	..	..	..	..	..	..	99	79	84	74	..	..
100	Belarus	..	..	..	..	..	..	..	..	..	94	86	91	96	..	..
101	Mauritius	97	98	96	99	99	99	100	100	100	87	88	89	84	78	..
102	Yugoslavia (former)	..	..	..	..	..	..	..	..	..	81	79	81	75	..	..
103	United Arab Emirates	95	..	..	77	93	22	99	..	..	98	90	90	90	..	81
104	Trinidad and Tobago	97	99	91	79	99	98	100	100	99	..	81	78	87	..	75
105	Uruguay	75	85	5	61	60	65	82	..	..	99	88	88	80	13	96
106	Lithuania	..	..	..	..	..	..	..	..	..	98	92	97	94	..	..
107	Panama	84	100	66	88	100	68	80x	95x	64x	91	81	83	83	27	70
108	Bulgaria	..	..	..	..	..	..	..	..	..	99	97	99	92	..	..
109	Sri Lanka	60	80	55	50	68	45	93x	..	..	86	91	91	89	51	76
110	Colombia	86	87	82	64	84	18	60	..	..	94	83	85	94	40	40
111	Slovakia	..	..	..	..	..	..	..	..	..	91	99	99	96	..	..
112	Chile	86	98	75	83	84	5	97	..	..	97	94	94	93	..	90
113	Malaysia	78	96	66	94	..	..	..	..	..	99	89	89	80	81	47
114	Costa Rica	93	100	86	97	100	94	80x	100x	63x	97	86	87	82	68	78
115	Poland	..	..	..	..	..	..	..	..	..	94	98	98	96	..	..
116	Hungary	..	..	..	..	..	..	..	..	..	99	100	100	100	..	..
117	Jamaica	100	100	100	89	100	80	90	..	..	99	91	93	72	50	10
118	Kuwait	..	100	..	..	100	..	100	..	..	3	98	98	93	44	10
119	Portugal	..	..	..	..	..	..	..	..	..	92	94	93	99	..	..
120	Cuba	98	100	91	92	100	68	98	99	96	97	99	97	93	98	80
121	United States	..	..	..	..	..	..	..	..	..	..	83	72	83	..	..
122	Czech Rep.	..	..	..	..	..	..	..	..	..	98	99	99	97	..	..
123	Greece	..	..	..	..	..	..	..	..	..	56	54	77	76	..	..
124	Belgium	..	..	..	..	..	..	..	..	..	..	85	100	77	..	..
125	Spain	..	..	..	..	..	..	..	..	..	..	84	85	83	..	..
126	France	..	..	..	..	..	..	..	..	..	78	89	92	76	..	..
127	Korea, Rep. of	93	100	76	100	100	100	100	100	100	94	97	95	89	..	..
128	Israel	..	..	..	..	..	..	..	..	..	..	92	91	96	..	..
129	Italy	..	..	..	..	..	..	..	..	..	6	95	98	50	..	..
130	New Zealand	97	100	82	..	..	..	..	..	..	20	81	68	82	..	..
131	Australia	..	..	..	..	..	..	..	..	..	..	95	72	86	..	..
132	Canada	..	..	..	..	..	..	..	..	..	85x	85x	85x	85x	..	..
133	Switzerland	..	..	..	..	..	..	..	..	..	..	89	95	83	..	..
134	United Kingdom	..	..	..	..	..	..	..	..	..	75	92	95	92	..	..
135	Austria	..	..	..	..	..	..	..	..	..	97	90	90	60	..	..
136	Netherlands	..	..	..	..	..	..	..	..	..	..	97	97	95	..	..
137	Norway	..	..	..	..	..	..	..	..	..	95	96	93	94	..	..
138	Germany	..	..	..	..	..	..	..	..	..	84	75	90	70	..	..
139	Ireland	..	..	..	..	..	..	..	..	..	..	65	63	78	..	..
140	Hong Kong	100	100	96	88	90	50	99x	..	..	99	82	81	75	..	..
141	Denmark	..	..	..	..	..	..	..	..	..	..	88	95	81	..	..
142	Japan	97	100	85	..	85	..	..	..	..	85	87	90	66	..	..
143	Singapore	100	100	..	99	99	..	100	100	..	99	89	92	89	..	..
144	Sweden	..	..	..	..	..	..	..	..	..	14	99	99	95	..	..
145	Finland	..	..	..	..	..	..	..	..	..	99	99	100	99	..	..

Countries listed in descending order of their 1993 under-five mortality rates (table 1).

Table 4: Education

		Adult literacy rate 1970 male	1970 female	1990 male	1990 female	No. of sets per 1000 population 1991 radio	television	Primary school enrolment ratio 1960 (gross) male	female	1986-92 (gross) male	female	1986-92 (net) male	female	% of primary school children reaching grade 5 1986-92	Secondary school enrolment ratio 1986-92 (gross) male	female
1	Niger	6	2	40	17	60	5	8	3	37	21	31	19	82	9	4
2	Angola	16	7	56	29	28	6	30	14	95	87	..	..	34	..	..
3	Sierra Leone	18	8	31	11	223	10	30	15	56	39	..	..	..	21	12
4	Mozambique	29	14	45	21	47	3	71	43	69	50	49	39	34	9	5
5	Afghanistan	13	2	44	14	107	8	14	2	32	17	25	14	43	11	6
6	Guinea-Bissau	13	6	50	24	40	..	35	15	77	42	58	32	20	9	4
7	Guinea	21	7	35	13	42	7	27	9	50	24	34	17	59	15	5
8	Malawi	42	18	65x	34x	220	..	50	26	72	60	50	47	46	5	3
9	Liberia	27	8	50	29	225	18	40	13	51x	28x	..	..	..	31x	12x
10	Mali	11	4	41	24	44	1	13	5	32	19	17	14	76	10	5
11	Somalia	5	1	36	14	37	12	6	2	15x	8x	11x	6x	..	9x	5x
12	Chad	20	2	42	18	243	1	29	4	89	41	52	23	76	12	3
13	Eritrea	..	..	..	..	..	..	..	..	..	..	..	..	..	..	..
14	Ethiopia	8	..	33x	16x	189	3	9	3	29	21	33	24	31	13	11
15	Zambia	66	37	81	65	81	26	61	40	101	92	83	80	..	25	14
16	Mauritania	..	..	47	21	144	23	12	3	63	48	..	..	77	19	10
17	Bhutan	..	..	51	25	16	..	5	..	31	19	..	..	..	7	2
18	Nigeria	35	14	62	40	173	33	54	31	79	62	..	..	65	24	17
19	Zaire	61	22	84	61	97	1	89	32	87	64	66	51	..	32	15
20	Uganda	52	30	62	35	109	10	39	18	78	64	58	51	..	16	8
21	Cambodia	..	23	48	22	112	8	..	..	..	..	..	..	..	..	..
22	Burundi	29	10	61	40	60	1	33	10	77	63	55	46	62	7	4
23	Central African Rep.	26	6	52	25	68	4	50	11	85	52	68	44	65	17	7
24	Burkina Faso	13	3	28	9	26	5	12	5	46	29	36	23	63	10	5
25	Ghana	43	18	70	51	268	15	58	31	84	69	..	..	69	47	29
26	Tanzania, U. Rep. of	48	18	62x	31x	25	2	33	16	70	68	50	50	79	6	4
27	Madagascar	56	43	88	73	200	20	74	57	93	91	64	63	38	18	18
28	Lesotho	49	74	..	..	32	6	73	109	97	116	62	77	65	21	31
29	Gabon	43	22	74	49	143	37	..	..	..	..	..	..	50	..	..
30	Benin	23	8	32	16	90	5	39	15	78	39	60	31	47	17	7
31	Lao Peo. Dem. Rep.	37	28	92x	76x	125	6	43	20	112	84	66	53	..	27	17
32	Rwanda	43	21	64	37	64	..	65	29	72	70	67	67	60	9	7
33	Pakistan	30	11	47	21	90	18	39	11	54	30	..	..	48	29	13
34	Yemen	14	3	53	26	27	27	..	..	111	43	..	..	..	47	10
35	Togo	27	7	56	31	211	6	64	25	134	87	89	62	70	35	12
36	Haiti	26x	17x	59	47	47	5	50	39	58	54	25	26	47	22	21
37	Sudan	28	6	43	12	250	77	29	11	56	43	..	..	94	25	20
38	Nepal	23	3	38	13	33	2	19	3	108	54	80	41	..	43	17
39	Bangladesh	36	12	47	22	43	5	80	31	83	71	74	64	47	25	12
40	India	47	20	62	34	79	35	83	44	112	84	..	..	62	54	32
41	Côte d'Ivoire	26	10	67	40	142	59	62	22	81	58	..	..	73	32	16
42	Senegal	18	5	52	25	114	36	37	18	68	49	55	41	88	21	11
43	Bolivia	68	46	85	71	625	103	70	43	89	81	85	78	60	37	31
44	Cameroon	47	19	66	43	145	24	77	37	109	93	82	71	66	32	23
45	Indonesia	66	42	88	75	146	59	78	58	119	114	100	96	83	49	41
46	Myanmar	85	57	89	72	82	2	60	53	107	100	..	..	..	25	23
47	Congo	50	19	70	44	113	6	..	..	..	..	..	..	72	..	..
48	Libyan Arab Jamahiriya	60	13	75	50	225	99	..	..	..	..	..	..	..	..	..
49	Papua New Guinea	39	24	65	38	73	2	24	15	76	65	78	66	69	15	10
50	Kenya	44	19	80	59	86	10	62	29	97	93	92x	89x	67	33	25
51	Turkmenistan	..	..	99x	97x	..	..	..	..	..	..	..	..	..	..	..
52	Turkey	69	34	90	69	161	175	90	58	115	110	..	..	98	60	40
53	Zimbabwe	63	47	74	60	84	26	82	65	120	118	..	..	94	54	42
54	Tajikistan	..	..	99x	97x	..	..	..	..	..	..	..	..	..	..	..
55	Namibia	..	..	..	..	127	21	..	..	112	126	..	..	53	36	47
56	Mongolia	87	74	..	..	132	40	80	80	96	100	..	..	..	87	96
57	Guatemala	51	37	63	47	66	52	48	39	84	73	..	..	..	20x	17x
58	Nicaragua	58	57	36x	33x	262	65	57	59	98	104	77	79	46	42	46
59	Iraq	50	18	70	49	215	72	94	36	120	102	100	87	72	59	37
60	South Africa	..	..	78x	75x	303	98	..	..	..	..	..	..	..	..	..
61	Algeria	39	11	70	46	234	74	55	37	103	88	94	83	95	66	53
62	Uzbekistan	..	..	98x	96x	..	..	..	..	..	..	..	..	..	..	..
63	Brazil	69	63	82	81	386	207	58	56	101x	97x	..	..	39	31x	36x
64	Peru	81	60	91	79	253	98	98	74	125x	120x	..	..	..	66x	60x
65	El Salvador	61	53	76	70	412	92	59	56	76	77	70	72	45	22	27
66	Egypt	50	20	63	34	326	116	79	52	109	93	..	..	91	90	73
67	Morocco	34	10	61	38	210	74	69	28	78	54	67	47	80	40	29
68	Philippines	84	81	94	93	138	44	98	93	113	111	100	100	75	71	75
69	Kyrgyzstan	..	..	98x	94x	..	..	..	..	..	..	..	..	..	..	..
70	Ecuador	75	68	90	84	317	84	82	75	119	117	..	..	67	55	57
71	Botswana	37	44	84	65	122	16	38	43	116	121	95	100	84	50	57
72	Honduras	55	50	75	71	386	73	68	67	102	107	88	93	..	..	..
73	Iran, Islamic Rep. of	40	17	64	43	231	63	59	28	118	105	100	93	90	66	49
74	Azerbaijan	..	..	99x	96x	..	..	..	..	..	..	..	..	..	..	..
75	Kazakhstan	..	..	99x	96x	..	..	..	..	..	..	..	..	..	..	..

		Adult literacy rate 1970		Adult literacy rate 1990		No. of sets per 1000 population 1991		Primary school enrolment ratio 1960 (gross)		1986-92 (gross)		1986-92 (net)		% of primary school children reaching grade 5 1986-92	Secondary school enrolment ratio 1986-92 (gross)	
		male	female	male	female	radio	television	male	female	male	female	male	female		male	female
76	Dominican Rep.	69	65	85	82	171	84	75	74	95	96	73	73	..	44x	57x
77	Viet Nam	..	..	92	84	104	41	103	74	106x	100x	..	..	..	44x	41x
78	China	..	..	87	68	182	31	131	90	127	118	99	94	86	56	45
79	Albania	..	..	..	..	176	87	102	86	100	101	..	..	98	84	74
80	Lebanon	79x	58x	88	73	833	325	112	105	115	110	..	..	..	62	64
81	Syrian Arab Rep.	60	20	78	51	255	60	89	39	115	103	100	94	92	56	43
82	Saudi Arabia	15	2	73	48	304	266	32	3	82	72	68	56	88	51	41
83	Moldova	..	..	99x	94x	..	..	..	..	..	..	..	..	..	..	..
84	Tunisia	44	17	74	56	199	79	88	43	123	110	100	93	88	51	42
85	Paraguay	85x	75x	92	88	171	50	106	94	111	108	97	97	70	30	31
86	Armenia	..	..	99x	98x	..	..	..	..	..	..	..	..	..	..	..
87	Thailand	86	72	95	91	191	114	97	88	92	88	..	..	88	34	32
88	Mexico	78	69	90	85	255	148	80	75	115	112	..	..	80	56	55
89	Korea, Dem. Peo. Rep.	..	..	..	..	119	15	..	..	108	100	..	..	..	..	..
90	Russian Federation	..	..	100x	98x	678x	..	..	..	..	..	..	..	..	..	..
91	Romania	96	91	99x	95x	199	196	101	95	90	90	..	..	90	81	80
92	Oman	..	..	..	..	637	728	..	..	104	96	84	79	96	61	53
93	Georgia	..	..	99x	98x	..	..	..	..	..	..	..	..	..	..	..
94	Jordan	64	29	89	70	256	80	..	..	96	98	90	92	100	63	62
95	Argentina	94	92	95	95	682	220	99	,99	108	115	..	..	..	67	74
96	Latvia	..	..	100x	99x	..	372	..	..	..	..	..	..	..	..	..
97	Ukraine	..	..	99x	97x	1177	487	..	..	..	..	..	..	..	..	..
98	Venezuela	79	71	87	90	447	162	98	99	98	100	90	92	86	29	40
99	Estonia	..	..	100x	100x	..	347	..	..	..	..	..	..	..	..	..
100	Belarus	..	..	99x	97x	306x	268x	..	..	..	..	..	..	98	..	..
101	Mauritius	77	59	85	75	359	217	96	90	104	108	87	90	98	52	56
102	Yugoslavia (former)	92	76	97	88	246s	198x	..	..	94	94	80x	79x	..	80	79
103	United Arab Emirates	24	7	58x	38x	325	107	..	..	117	114	100	100	89	65	73
104	Trinidad and Tobago	95	89	96x	93x	492	315	111	108	96	96	90	90	89	80	82
105	Uruguay	93x	93x	97	96	637	231	117	117	109	107	91	92	94	61x	62x
106	Lithuania	..	..	99x	98x	..	374	..	..	..	..	..	..	82	57	62
107	Panama	81	81	89	88	224	166	89	86	109	105	91	92	91	70	73
108	Bulgaria	94	89	..	..	442	252	94	92	93	91	82	81	95	71	77
109	Sri Lanka	85	69	93	83	197	35x	107	95	110	106	..	..	56	51	60
110	Colombia	79	76	87	86	177	116	74	74	110	112	..	..			
111	Slovakia	..	..	..	..	..	..	..	..	..	..	..	..	98	70	75
112	Chile	90	88	93	93	344	209	87	86	99	97	88	86	98	57	59
113	Malaysia	71	48	86	70	430	149	108	79	93	93	..	..	84	42	45
114	Costa Rica	88	87	93	93	257	140	94	92	103	102	87	88	99	82	86
115	Poland	98	97	99x	98x	433	295	110	107	99	97	97	96			
116	Hungary	98	98	99x	98x	596	412	103	100	89	89	85	86	98	81	81
117	Jamaica	96	97	98	99	420	131	78	79	105	108	99	100	96	59	66
118	Kuwait	65	42	77	67	343	283	132	99	56	55	46	43	..	51	51
119	Portugal	78	65	89	81	228	187	132	129	120	115	97	98	..	63	74
120	Cuba	86	87	95	93	345	163	109	110	103	102	97	97	91	81	94
121	United States	99	99	..	..	2118	814	..	..	104	104	98	99	..	90	90
122	Czech Rep.	..	..	..	..	..	..	..	..	..	..	..	..	..	..	..
123	Greece	93	76	98	89	421	197	104	101	97	98	93	94	98	99	97
124	Belgium	99	99	..	..	769	451	111	108	98	100	94	96	..	102	103
125	Spain	93	87	97	93	310	400	106	116	109	108	100	100	97	104	113
126	France	99	98	..	..	888	407	144	143	108	106	100	100	96	99	104
127	Korea, Rep. of	94	81	99	93	1001	208	108	94	103	106	100	100	100	90	91
128	Israel	93	83	95x	89x	470	269	99	97	93	96	..	..	100	82	89
129	Italy	95	93	98	96	791	421	112	109	94	94	..	..	100	76	76
130	New Zealand	..	..	..	..	927	443	110	106	104	103	100	99	94	83	85
131	Australia	..	..	..	..	1268	480	103	103	107	107	98	98	99	81	83
132	Canada	..	..	..	..	1029	639	108	105	108	106	99	98	96	104	104
133	Switzerland	..	..	..	..	842	406	118	118	103	104	95	95	100	94	88
134	United Kingdom	..	..	..	..	1143	434	92	92	104	105	97	98	..	85	88
135	Austria	..	..	..	..	617	478	106	104	103	102	90	91	100	107	100
136	Netherlands	..	..	..	..	907	485	105	104	100	103	93	97	..	98	95
137	Norway	..	..	..	..	794	423	100	100	100	100	99	99	100	103	104
138	Germany	..	..	..	..	876	556	..	..	105	105	89	90	..	99	96
139	Ireland	..	..	..	..	630	276x	107	112	103	103	90	91	99	96	105
140	Hong Kong	..	..	90x	64x	667	278	88	72	105	105	95x	95x	..	73	77
141	Denmark	..	..	..	..	1031	536	103	103	96	96	96	96	99	107	110
142	Japan	99	99	..	..	907	613	103	102	102	..	100	100	100	96	98
143	Singapore	92	55	92x	74x	646	378	120	101	110	107	100	100	100	70	71
144	Sweden	..	..	..	..	877	468	95	96	100	100	100	100	100	89	93
145	Finland	..	..	..	..	997	501	100	95	99	99	..	..	100	107	133

Countries listed in descending order of their 1993 under-five mortality rates (table 1).

73

Table 5: Demographic indicators

		Population (millions) 1993 under 16	Population (millions) 1993 under 5	Population annual growth rate (%) 1965-80	Population annual growth rate (%) 1980-93	Crude death rate 1960	Crude death rate 1993	Crude birth rate 1960	Crude birth rate 1993	Life expectancy 1960	Life expectancy 1993	Total fertility rate 1993	% of population urbanized 1993	Average annual growth rate of urban population (%) 1965-80	Average annual growth rate of urban population (%) 1980-93
1	Niger	4.3	1.7	2.8	3.3	29	19	53	51	35	47	7.1	22	7.2	7.1
2	Angola	5.1	2.0	2.0	3.0	31	19	50	51	33	47	7.1	31	5.5	6.0
3	Sierra Leone	2.1	0.8	2.0	2.5	33	21	48	48	32	43	6.5	35	5.1	5.1
4	Mozambique	7.2	2.8	2.5	1.8	26	18	47	45	37	47	6.5	32	9.5	8.6
5	Afghanistan	8.7	3.7	1.9	1.9	30	22	52	52	33	44	6.8	19	5.3	3.6
6	Guinea-Bissau	0.4	0.2	2.8	2.0	29	21	40	43	34	44	5.8	21	3.9	3.8
7	Guinea	3.1	1.2	1.6	2.7	31	20	53	50	34	45	7.0	28	4.9	5.7
8	Malawi	5.5	2.2	2.9	4.2	28	21	54	54	38	44	7.5	13	7.1	6.8
9	Liberia	1.4	0.5	3.0	3.2	25	14	50	47	41	56	6.8	49	6.1	5.8
10	Mali	5.0	2.0	2.2	3.0	29	19	52	50	35	46	7.1	26	4.8	5.6
11	Somalia	4.7	1.9	3.1	2.7	28	18	50	50	36	47	7.0	25	3.9	3.7
12	Chad	2.7	1.1	2.0	2.3	30	18	46	44	35	48	5.9	35	7.5	6.4
13	Eritrea	1.6	0.6	..	..	..	16	..	42	..	47	5.8	..	..	..
14	Ethiopia	24.8	10.0	2.4	2.6	28	18	51	49	36	47	7.0	13	4.5	4.3
15	Zambia	4.5	1.7	3.1	3.4	22	18	50	46	42	44	6.3	43	6.6	3.9
16	Mauritania	1.0	0.4	2.3	2.7	28	17	48	46	35	48	6.5	51	10.1	7.1
17	Bhutan	0.7	0.3	1.9	2.2	26	16	42	40	37	49	5.8	6	4.2	5.4
18	Nigeria	59.0	22.5	3.2	3.2	24	14	52	45	40	53	6.4	38	6.3	5.8
19	Zaire	20.6	8.1	2.9	3.2	23	15	47	47	41	52	6.7	29	3.5	3.3
20	Uganda	9.8	3.9	3.3	2.9	21	21	50	51	43	42	7.2	12	5.3	5.4
21	Cambodia	3.9	1.5	0.4	2.5	21	14	45	39	42	51	4.5	12	0.0	3.9
22	Burundi	2.9	1.1	1.7	2.9	23	17	46	46	41	48	6.7	6	6.1	5.2
23	Central African Rep.	1.5	0.6	2.1	2.6	26	18	43	44	39	47	6.2	49	4.5	4.6
24	Burkina Faso	4.6	1.8	2.3	2.6	28	17	49	47	36	48	6.5	18	5.5	8.4
25	Ghana	7.8	2.9	2.1	3.3	19	12	48	42	45	56	5.9	35	3.3	4.3
26	Tanzania, U. Rep. of	14.4	5.7	3.0	3.4	23	15	51	48	41	51	6.8	23	9.9	6.8
27	Madagascar	6.3	2.4	2.5	3.2	24	13	48	45	41	56	6.6	26	5.1	5.9
28	Lesotho	0.8	0.3	2.2	2.6	24	10	43	34	43	61	4.7	22	7.1	6.4
29	Gabon	0.5	0.2	3.3	3.6	24	16	31	43	41	54	5.4	48	6.7	5.9
30	Benin	2.5	1.0	2.4	2.9	33	18	47	49	35	46	7.1	40	8.3	4.9
31	Lao Peo. Dem. Rep.	2.1	0.8	1.8	2.8	23	15	45	45	40	51	6.6	21	5.1	6.1
32	Rwanda	4.0	1.6	3.2	3.2	22	18	50	52	42	46	8.4	6	6.8	4.9
33	Pakistan	58.8	22.0	2.7	3.1	23	10	49	40	43	59	6.1	34	3.8	4.5
34	Yemen	6.7	2.6	2.3	3.5	28	13	53	48	36	53	7.1	32	6.3	7.1
35	Togo	1.9	0.7	3.2	3.0	26	13	48	44	39	55	6.5	30	7.9	5.1
36	Haiti	2.9	1.0	1.7	1.9	23	12	42	35	42	57	4.8	30	3.7	3.9
37	Sudan	12.9	4.8	2.8	2.9	25	14	47	42	39	52	6.0	24	5.6	4.3
38	Nepal	9.6	3.4	2.4	2.7	26	13	46	37	38	54	5.4	13	6.6	7.8
39	Bangladesh	52.5	18.7	2.8	2.5	22	13	47	38	40	53	4.7	18	6.7	6.3
40	India	335.4	113.4	2.2	2.0	21	10	43	29	44	61	3.8	26	3.6	3.0
41	Côte d'Ivoire	6.8	2.7	4.0	3.8	25	15	53	50	39	51	7.4	42	6.7	5.3
42	Senegal	3.8	1.4	2.8	2.8	27	16	50	43	37	49	6.0	41	3.4	3.9
43	Bolivia	3.3	1.1	2.5	2.5	22	9	46	34	43	61	4.5	53	3.2	3.9
44	Cameroon	5.8	2.2	2.6	2.9	24	12	44	41	39	56	5.7	43	6.9	5.3
45	Indonesia	70.9	23.3	2.3	2.0	23	8	44	26	41	63	3.1	31	4.6	4.5
46	Myanmar	17.7	6.3	2.2	2.1	21	11	42	32	44	58	4.1	26	3.1	2.7
47	Congo	1.2	0.5	2.7	2.9	23	15	45	44	42	51	6.2	42	3.4	4.2
48	Libyan Arab Jamahiriya	2.4	0.9	4.2	3.9	19	8	49	42	47	63	6.3	85	10.4	5.4
49	Papua New Guinea	1.8	0.6	2.4	2.3	23	11	44	33	41	56	4.8	17	8.6	4.3
50	Kenya	13.2	4.9	3.6	3.5	22	10	53	44	45	59	6.2	26	7.7	7.2
51	Turkmenistan	1.7	0.6	..	..	..	8	..	36	..	66	4.5	..	..	..
52	Turkey	21.7	7.7	2.4	2.3	18	7	45	28	50	67	3.4	66	4.0	5.4
53	Zimbabwe	5.1	1.9	3.1	3.3	20	11	53	40	45	56	5.3	31	6.0	5.8
54	Tajikistan	2.8	1.0	..	..	..	6	..	41	..	69	5.3	32	..	..
55	Namibia	0.7	0.3	2.7	3.0	22	11	45	42	42	59	6.0	30	4.8	5.1
56	Mongolia	1.0	0.4	2.8	2.7	18	8	43	34	47	64	4.6	60	4.2	3.8
57	Guatemala	4.7	1.7	2.8	2.9	19	8	49	38	46	65	5.3	41	3.4	3.5
58	Nicaragua	2.0	0.7	3.1	3.0	19	7	51	40	47	67	5.0	62	4.6	4.1
59	Iraq	9.2	3.4	3.3	3.3	20	7	49	39	48	66	5.7	74	5.0	4.2
60	South Africa	16.4	5.6	2.7	2.5	17	8	42	31	49	63	4.1	50	2.8	2.8
61	Algeria	12.1	4.0	3.0	2.8	20	7	51	34	47	66	4.8	54	4.0	4.6
62	Uzbekistan	9.6	3.4	..	..	..	6	..	34	..	69	4.3	41	..	..
63	Brazil	55.3	17.2	2.4	2.0	13	7	43	23	55	66	2.7	77	4.3	3.2
64	Peru	8.8	2.9	2.7	2.2	19	8	47	29	48	65	3.5	71	4.2	2.9
65	El Salvador	2.4	0.8	2.7	1.5	16	7	49	33	50	67	4.0	46	3.2	2.3
66	Egypt	22.9	7.7	2.2	2.4	21	9	45	31	46	62	4.1	44	2.7	2.5
67	Morocco	11.2	3.9	2.5	2.5	21	8	50	32	47	64	4.3	48	4.2	3.7
68	Philippines	27.4	9.3	2.8	2.4	15	7	46	30	53	65	3.9	45	3.9	3.8
69	Kyrgyzstan	1.8	0.6	..	..	..	8	..	30	..	66	3.9	83	..	..
70	Ecuador	4.6	1.5	3.0	2.5	15	7	46	29	53	67	3.6	59	4.6	4.3
71	Botswana	0.6	0.2	3.3	3.1	20	9	52	38	46	61	5.0	29	12.5	8.1
72	Honduras	2.6	0.9	3.1	3.3	19	7	51	37	46	66	4.9	46	5.4	5.2
73	Iran, Islamic Rep. of	30.6	11.2	3.1	3.7	21	7	47	40	50	67	5.9	59	4.9	5.0
74	Azerbaijan	2.6	0.9	..	..	..	6	..	26	..	71	3.2	54	..	..
75	Kazakhstan	5.6	1.8	..	..	..	8	..	21	..	69	2.7	57	..	..

		Population (millions) 1993		Population annual growth rate (%)		Crude death rate		Crude birth rate		Life expectancy		Total fertility rate 1993	% of population urbanized 1993	Average annual growth rate of urban population (%)	
		under 16	under 5	1965-80	1980-93	1960	1993	1960	1993	1960	1993			1965-80	1980-93
76	Dominican Rep.	3.0	1.0	2.7	2.2	16	6	50	28	52	68	3.3	63	5.1	3.9
77	Viet Nam	28.2	9.4	2.2	2.1	23	8	41	29	44	64	3.8	20	3.3	2.6
78	China	348.4	120.2	2.1	1.5	19	7	37	21	47	71	2.2	29	2.6	4.4
79	Albania	1.1	0.4	2.4	1.7	10	5	41	23	62	73	2.7	37	2.9	2.3
80	Lebanon	1.1	0.4	1.4	0.6	14	7	43	27	60	69	3.1	86	4.1	1.9
81	Syrian Arab Rep.	6.9	2.6	3.3	3.5	18	6	47	42	50	67	6.1	52	4.3	4.3
82	Saudi Arabia	7.3	2.7	4.5	4.3	23	5	49	36	44	69	6.3	79	8.1	5.7
83	Moldova	1.4	0.4	..	..	..	10	..	16	..	68	2.5	47	..	..
84	Tunisia	3.3	1.1	2.1	2.3	19	6	47	27	48	68	3.4	58	3.8	3.3
85	Paraguay	2.0	0.7	2.9	3.0	9	6	43	33	64	67	4.3	49	3.8	4.3
86	Armenia	1.1	0.4	..	..	..	7	..	23	..	72	3.0	68	..	..
87	Thailand	18.4	5.6	2.8	1.5	15	6	44	20	52	69	2.2	24	4.7	4.2
88	Mexico	35.1	11.7	3.0	2.3	13	5	45	28	57	70	3.1	74	4.2	3.1
89	Korea, Dem. Peo. Rep.	7.0	2.6	2.6	1.8	13	5	42	24	54	71	2.4	61	4.1	2.3
90	Russian Federation	35.6	10.1	..	..	..	12	..	12	..	69	1.8	74	..	..
91	Romania	5.7	1.8	1.0	0.4	9	11	20	16	65	70	2.1	55	2.8	1.3
92	Oman	0.8	0.3	3.7	4.2	28	5	51	40	40	70	6.7	12	7.6	8.0
93	Georgia	1.4	0.4	..	..	..	9	..	15	..	73	2.1	56	..	..
94	Jordan	2.0	0.8	2.7	3.2	23	5	50	39	47	68	5.7	70	4.4	4.5
95	Argentina	10.3	3.2	1.6	1.3	9	9	24	20	65	71	2.8	87	2.1	1.7
96	Latvia	0.6	0.2	0.7	0.4	10	12	16	14	70	71	2.0	72	1.6	0.8
97	Ukraine	11.5	3.3	..	..	..	13	..	12	..	70	1.8	67	..	..
98	Venezuela	7.8	2.5	3.4	2.4	10	5	45	26	60	70	3.1	92	4.6	3.2
99	Estonia	0.4	0.1	0.9	0.5	11	12	16	14	69	72	2.1	73	1.7	0.8
100	Belarus	2.5	0.7	..	..	..	11	..	13	..	71	1.9	66	..	..
101	Mauritius	0.3	0.1	1.7	1.1	10	7	44	18	59	70	2.0	41	2.6	0.7
102	Yugoslavia (former)	5.7	1.7	0.9	0.6	10	9	24	14	63	72	1.9	59	3.4	2.6
103	United Arab Emirates	0.5	0.2	13.0	4.0	19	4	46	21	53	71	4.5	83	15.6	5.1
104	Trinidad and Tobago	0.5	0.1	1.3	1.3	9	6	38	23	63	71	2.7	66	1.2	1.6
105	Uruguay	0.8	0.3	0.5	0.6	10	10	22	17	68	72	2.3	90	0.9	1.0
106	Lithuania	0.9	0.3	1.0	0.7	8	10	21	15	69	73	2.0	71	3.0	1.8
107	Panama	0.9	0.3	2.6	2.1	10	5	41	25	61	73	2.8	54	3.3	2.7
108	Bulgaria	1.9	0.6	0.5	0.1	9	12	18	13	68	72	1.8	70	2.4	1.0
109	Sri Lanka	6.0	1.8	1.9	1.5	9	6	36	21	62	72	2.5	22	2.4	1.6
110	Colombia	12.3	3.9	2.4	1.9	12	6	45	24	57	69	2.6	72	3.6	2.8
111	Slovakia	1.4	0.4	..	..	..	10	..	15	..	72	2.0	..	..	..
112	Chile	4.5	1.5	1.7	1.7	13	6	37	22	57	72	2.7	85	2.6	2.0
113	Malaysia	7.7	2.7	2.5	2.6	15	5	44	28	54	71	3.6	46	4.4	4.7
114	Costa Rica	1.2	0.4	2.9	2.8	10	4	47	26	62	76	3.1	49	3.7	3.7
115	Poland	10.0	2.8	0.8	0.6	8	10	24	14	67	72	2.1	63	1.8	1.2
116	Hungary	2.2	0.6	0.4	-0.2	10	14	16	12	68	70	1.8	66	1.9	1.0
117	Jamaica	0.8	0.3	1.3	1.2	9	6	39	22	63	74	2.3	54	2.7	2.3
118	Kuwait	0.8	0.3	7.1	2.2	10	2	44	28	60	75	3.7	96	8.1	2.7
119	Portugal	2.1	0.6	0.4	0.1	11	10	24	12	63	75	1.5	35	1.8	1.5
120	Cuba	2.6	0.9	1.5	0.9	9	7	31	17	64	76	1.9	75	2.6	1.7
121	United States	59.7	19.7	1.1	1.0	9	9	23	16	70	76	2.1	76	1.2	1.2
122	Czech Rep.	2.3	0.7	..	..	..	11	..	13	..	72	1.9	..	..	..
123	Greece	2.0	0.5	0.8	0.4	8	10	19	10	69	78	1.5	64	2.1	1.2
124	Belgium	1.9	0.6	0.3	0.1	12	11	17	12	70	76	1.7	97	0.4	0.2
125	Spain	7.6	2.1	1.1	0.3	9	9	21	11	69	78	1.4	80	2.2	1.0
126	France	12.2	3.8	0.7	0.5	12	10	18	13	70	77	1.8	73	1.3	0.4
127	Korea, Rep. of	11.5	3.4	1.9	1.2	14	6	43	16	54	71	1.8	75	5.7	3.4
128	Israel	1.7	0.6	2.8	2.6	6	7	27	21	69	77	2.8	92	3.4	2.9
129	Italy	10.0	2.9	0.5	0.2	10	10	18	10	69	77	1.3	70	1.0	0.6
130	New Zealand	0.9	0.3	1.1	0.9	9	8	26	17	71	76	2.1	84	1.5	0.9
131	Australia	4.1	1.3	1.7	1.5	9	8	22	15	71	77	1.9	85	1.9	1.4
132	Canada	6.2	1.9	1.3	1.1	8	8	26	14	71	77	1.8	78	1.6	1.3
133	Switzerland	1.2	0.4	0.5	0.6	10	10	18	13	71	78	1.7	63	1.0	1.4
134	United Kingdom	11.9	3.9	0.2	0.2	12	11	17	14	71	76	1.9	89	0.4	0.2
135	Austria	1.5	0.4	0.3	0.3	12	11	18	12	69	76	1.5	60	0.8	0.9
136	Netherlands	3.0	1.0	0.9	0.6	8	9	21	14	73	77	1.7	89	1.2	0.6
137	Norway	0.9	0.3	0.6	0.4	9	11	18	15	73	77	2.0	76	2.0	1.0
138	Germany	14.6	4.6	0.2	0.2	12	11	17	11	70	76	1.5	86	0.6	0.5
139	Ireland	1.0	0.3	1.1	0.2	12	9	21	14	70	75	2.1	58	2.0	0.5
140	Hong Kong	1.2	0.4	2.1	1.1	7	6	35	13	66	78	1.5	95	2.5	1.4
141	Denmark	0.9	0.3	0.5	0.1	9	12	17	13	72	76	1.7	85	1.0	0.2
142	Japan	23.4	6.8	1.1	0.5	8	8	18	11	68	79	1.7	78	1.9	0.7
143	Singapore	0.7	0.2	1.7	1.1	8	6	38	16	64	75	1.8	100	1.7	1.1
144	Sweden	1.7	0.6	0.5	0.3	10	11	15	14	73	78	2.1	84	1.0	0.5
145	Finland	1.0	0.3	0.3	0.4	9	10	19	13	68	76	1.8	60	2.4	0.4

Countries listed in descending order of their 1993 under-five mortality rates (table 1).

Table 6: Economic indicators

		GNP per capita (US$) 1992	GNP per capita average annual growth rate (%) 1965-80	GNP per capita average annual growth rate (%) 1980-92	Rate of inflation (%) 1980-92	% of population below absolute poverty level 1980-89 urban	% of population below absolute poverty level 1980-89 rural	% of central government expenditure allocated to (1986-92) health	% of central government expenditure allocated to (1986-92) education	% of central government expenditure allocated to (1986-92) defence	ODA inflow in millions US$ 1992	ODA inflow as a % of recipient GNP 1992	Debt service as a % of exports of goods and services 1970	Debt service as a % of exports of goods and services 1992
1	Niger	280	-2.5	-4.3	2	..	35x	..	..	..	362	15	4	2
2	Angola	610x	..	6.1x	..	..	..	6x	15x	34x	322	..	..	6
3	Sierra Leone	160	0.7	-1.4	61	..	65x	10	13	10	134	18	11	3x
4	Mozambique	60	..	-3.6	38	50	67	5x	10x	35x	1393	135	..	7
5	Afghanistan	280x	0.6	..	..	18x	36x	..	..	..	174	..	..	..
6	Guinea-Bissau	220	-2.7	1.6	59	..	..	1	3	4	107	49	..	88
7	Guinea	510	1.3	..	..	..	..	..	11x	29x	463	15	..	12
8	Malawi	210	3.2	-0.1	15	25	85	7	9	5	521	27	8	18
9	Liberia	450x	0.5	5.2x	..	..	23x	5	11	9	118	..	8	..
10	Mali	310	2.1x	-2.7	4	27x	48x	2	9	8	439	16	1	2x
11	Somalia	150x	-0.1	-1.8x	50	40x	70x	1x	2x	38x	577	..	2	7x
12	Chad	220	-1.9	3.4	1	30x	56x	8x	8x	..	248	20	4	4
13	Eritrea	110	..	..	..	..	..	..	..	..	..	..	..	..
14	Ethiopia	110	0.4	-1.9	3	60	65	3	11	..	1301	21	11	14
15	Zambia	290	-1.2	-2.9x	48	25	..	7	9	..	1016	39	6	21
16	Mauritania	530	-0.1	-0.8	8	..	..	4x	23x	..	210	19	3	15x
17	Bhutan	180	..	6.3	9	..	..	5	11	..	63	24	..	8x
18	Nigeria	320	4.2	-0.4	19	..	..	1	3	3	265	1	4	30
19	Zaire	230x	-1.3	-1.6x	61xx	..	80x	4x	6x	14x	269	..	4	6x
20	Uganda	170	-2.2	3.3x	107xx	..	..	2x	15x	26x	718	24	3	22
21	Cambodia	200x	..	..	..	..	..	..	..	..	148	..	..	..
22	Burundi	210	2.4	1.3	5	55x	85x	4x	16x	16x	316	26	2	36
23	Central African Rep.	410	0.8	-1.5	5	..	91	..	..	..	179	14	5	8
24	Burkina Faso	300	1.7	1.0	4	..	..	5	14	18	444	15	7	8x
25	Ghana	450	-0.8	-0.1	39	59	37	9	26	3	626	9	6	17
26	Tanzania, U. Rep. of	110	0.8	0.0	25	..	..	6x	8x	16x	1344	52	5	30
27	Madagascar	230	-0.4	-2.4	16	50x	50x	7	17	8	359	13	4	16
28	Lesotho	590	6.8	-0.5	13	50x	55x	11	22	6	142	13	5	5
29	Gabon	4450	5.6	-3.7	2	..	..	..	..	..	69	1	6	13
30	Benin	410	-0.3	-0.7	2	..	..	6x	31x	17x	269	13	2	4
31	Lao Peo. Dem. Rep.	250	..	1.2x	..	..	..	..	..	..	173	16	..	9x
32	Rwanda	250	1.6	-0.6	4	30	90x	5x	26x	..	352	19	1	14x
33	Pakistan	420	1.8	3.1	7	32x	29x	1	2x	28x	1169	2	24	17
34	Yemen	520	..	..	..	..	..	5	21	21	262	4	..	7x
35	Togo	390	1.7	-1.8	4	42x	..	5	20	11	225	14	3	4
36	Haiti	370	0.9	-2.4x	7x	65	80	..	..	..	106	4	59	3x
37	Sudan	420x	0.8	-2.4x	43	..	85x	..	..	..	608	..	11	5
38	Nepal	170	..	2.0	9	55x	61x	5	11	6	467	14	3	11
39	Bangladesh	220	-0.3	1.8	9	86x	86x	5x	11x	10x	1728	7	..	14
40	India	310	1.5	3.1	9	29	33	2	2	17	2435	1	22	21
41	Côte d'Ivoire	670	2.8	-4.7	2	30	26	4x	..	..	763	9	7	15
42	Senegal	780	-0.5	0.1	5	..	..	..	..	..	673	11	3	8
43	Bolivia	680	1.7	-1.5	221	..	..	3	19	13	679	13	11	28
44	Cameroon	820	2.4	-1.5	4	15x	40x	3	12	7	727	7	3	7
45	Indonesia	670	5.2	4.0	8	20	16	2	9	8	2080	2	7	20
46	Myanmar	220x	1.6	..	15	40x	40x	7	16	22	126	..	12	11x
47	Congo	1030	2.7	-0.8	1	..	..	..	..	..	115	5	12	9
48	Libyan Arab Jamahiriya	5310x	0.0	-9.2x	0xx	..	..	..	..	..	22	..	..	..
49	Papua New Guinea	950	..	0.0	5	10x	75x	9	15	5	483	13	1	9
50	Kenya	310	3.1	0.2	9	10x	55x	5	20	10	780	9	6	14
51	Turkmenistan	1230	..	0.7x	..	..	..	..	..	..	..	..	..	..
52	Turkey	1980	3.6	2.9	46	..	..	3	18	10	323	0	22	26
53	Zimbabwe	570	1.7	-0.9	14	..	..	8x	..	17x	735	12	2	25
54	Tajikistan	490	..	-0.1x	..	..	..	..	..	..	..	..	..	..
55	Namibia	1610	..	-1.0	12	..	..	10	22	7	140	6	..	..
56	Mongolia	780x	..	..	-1x	..	..	..	..	..	105	..	..	17
57	Guatemala	980	3.0	-1.5	17	17	51	10	20	13	210	2	7	24
58	Nicaragua	340	-0.7	-5.3	656	21x	19x	11x	9x	50x	662	50	11	25
59	Iraq	1500x	..	..	..	..	..	..	..	..	187	..	..	..
60	South Africa	2670	3.2	0.1	14	..	..	..	..	..	..	..	..	..
61	Algeria	1840	4.2	-0.5	11	20x	..	..	..	..	412	1	4	69
62	Uzbekistan	850	..	0.8x	..	..	..	..	..	..	..	..	..	..
63	Brazil	2770	6.3	0.4	370	9	34	7	3	4	-236	0	13	16
64	Peru	950	0.8	-2.8	312	46	83	6	21	18	419	2	12	17
65	El Salvador	1170	1.5	0.0	17	20	32	8	14	21	399	6	4	12
66	Egypt	640	2.8	1.8	13	34	34	3	13	13	3538	10	38	12
67	Morocco	1030	2.7	1.4	7	28x	45x	3	17	15	996	4	9	23x
68	Philippines	770	3.2	-1.0	14	52	64	4	16	11	1738	4	8	25
69	Kyrgyzstan	820	..	2.1x	..	..	..	..	..	..	..	..	..	..
70	Ecuador	1070	5.4	-0.3	40	40	65	11	18	13	249	2	9	22
71	Botswana	2790	9.9	6.1	13	40	55	5	21	13	113	3	1	3x
72	Honduras	580	1.1	-0.3	8	31	70	..	..	7x	355	11	3	32
73	Iran, Islamic Rep. of	2200	2.9	-1.4	16	..	..	8	21	10	169	0	..	1
74	Azerbaijan	740	..	0.4x	..	..	..	..	..	..	..	..	..	..
75	Kazakhstan	1680	..	0.9x	..	..	..	..	..	..	..	..	..	..

#	Country	GNP per capita (US$) 1992	GNP per capita average annual growth rate (%) 1965-80	GNP per capita average annual growth rate (%) 1980-92	Rate of inflation (%) 1980-92	% of population below absolute poverty level 1980-89 urban	% of population below absolute poverty level 1980-89 rural	% of central government expenditure allocated to (1986-92) health	% of central government expenditure allocated to (1986-92) education	% of central government expenditure allocated to (1986-92) defence	ODA inflow in millions US$ 1992	ODA inflow as a % of recipient GNP 1992	Debt service as a % of exports of goods and services 1970	Debt service as a % of exports of goods and services 1992
76	Dominican Rep.	1050	3.8	-0.5	25	45x	43x	14	10	5	62	1	4	11
77	Viet Nam	240x	..	..	..	..	..	..	..	..	586	..	..	..
78	China	470	4.1	7.6	7	..	13	..	..	8x	3065	1	..	9
79	Albania	790x	..	..	..	..	..	..	..	..	389	..	..	2
80	Lebanon	2150x	..	..	..	..	..	..	..	..	81	..	..	3
81	Syrian Arab Rep.	1160	5.1	-1.4x	16	..	..	2	7	32	163	1	11	25x
82	Saudi Arabia	7510	4.0x	-3.3	-2	..	..	..	..	..	80	0	..	..
83	Moldova	1300	..	1.8x	..	..	..	..	..	..	..	..	..	1
84	Tunisia	1720	4.7	1.3	7	20x	15x	6	17	6	407	3	20	19
85	Paraguay	1380	4.1	-0.7	25	19x	50x	4	13	13	99	2	12	40
86	Armenia	780	..	2.1x	..	..	..	..	..	..	..	..	..	..
87	Thailand	1840	4.4	6.0	4	10	25	7	20	17	789	1	3	5x
88	Mexico	3470	3.6	-0.2	62	..	..	2	14	2	317	0	24	33
89	Korea, Dem. Peo. Rep.	970x	..	..	..	..	..	..	..	..	12	..	..	..
90	Russian Federation	2510	..	1.3x	..	..	..	..	..	..	..	..	..	..
91	Romania	1130	..	-1.1	13	..	..	9	10	10	..	..	..	3
92	Oman	6480	9.0	4.1	-3	..	..	5	11	35	54	1	..	12x
93	Georgia	850	..	2.2x	..	..	..	..	..	..	..	..	..	..
94	Jordan	1120	5.8x	-5.4	5	14x	17x	5	15	21	379	9	4	18
95	Argentina	6050	1.7	-0.9	402	..	..	3	10	10	286	0	22	24
96	Latvia	1930	..	0.2	15	..	..	..	..	..	..	..	..	..
97	Ukraine	1820	..	2.3x	..	..	..	..	..	..	..	..	..	0
98	Venezuela	2910	2.3	-0.8	23	..	..	10	20	6x	40	0	..	11
99	Estonia	2760	..	-2.3	20	..	..	..	..	..	..	..	..	1
100	Belarus	2930	..	3.3x	..	..	..	..	..	..	..	..	..	..
101	Mauritius	2700	3.7	5.6	9	12x	12x	9	15	2	47	2	3	7
102	Yugoslavia (former)	3060x	5.2	-1.4x	123x	..	..	..	..	53	1148	..	10	12x
103	United Arab Emirates	22020	..	-4.3	1	..	..	7	15	44	-8	..	..	..
104	Trinidad and Tobago	3940	3.1	-2.6	4	..	39x	..	..	..	8	0	5	19
105	Uruguay	3340	2.5	-1.0	66	22	..	4	7	9	70	1	22	16
106	Lithuania	1310	..	-1.0	21	..	..	..	..	..	..	..	..	..
107	Panama	2420	2.8	-1.2	2	21x	30x	21	17	5	157	3	8	22
108	Bulgaria	1330	..	1.2	12	..	..	5	6	6	..	..	..	4
109	Sri Lanka	540	2.8	2.6	11	..	..	5	8	9	658	7	11	10
110	Colombia	1330	3.7	1.4	25	32	70	..	..	..	240	1	12	32
111	Slovakia	1930	..	..	..	..	..	..	..	..	..	..	..	..
112	Chile	2730	0.0	3.7	21	12	20	6	10	8	137	0	19	11
113	Malaysia	2790	4.7	3.2	2	13	38	5	19	12	213	0	4	5
114	Costa Rica	1960	3.3	0.8	23	8	20	32	19	2	136	2	10	18
115	Poland	1910	..	0.1	68	..	..	..	..	..	..	..	..	8
116	Hungary	2970	5.1	0.2	12	..	..	8x	3x	4x	..	..	..	31
117	Jamaica	1340	-0.1	0.2	22	..	80	7x	11x	8x	126	4	3	20
118	Kuwait	16150x	0.6x	-2.2x	-3xx	..	..	7	14	20	3	..	..	..
119	Portugal	7450	4.6	3.1	17	..	..	..	..	6x	..	..	7	20x
120	Cuba	1170x	..	..	..	..	..	23x	10x	..	30	..	..	..
121	United States	23240	1.8	1.7	4	..	..	14	2	22	..	..	..	..
122	Czech Rep.	2450	..	..	..	..	..	..	..	..	..	..	..	..
123	Greece	7290	4.8	1.0	18	..	..	..	..	..	46	0	9	..
124	Belgium	20880	3.6	2.0	4	..	..	12x	2x	5x	..	..	..	..
125	Spain	13970	4.1	2.9	9	..	..	14	6	5	..	..	..	..
126	France	22260	3.7	1.7	5	..	..	15x	7x	7x	..	..	..	..
127	Korea, Rep. of	6790	7.3	8.5	6	18x	11x	1	16	22	4	0	20	5
128	Israel	13220	3.7	1.9	79	..	..	4	10	22	2066	3	3	..
129	Italy	20460	3.2	2.2	9	..	..	11x	8x	4x	..	..	..	..
130	New Zealand	12300	1.7	0.6	9	..	..	12	12	4	..	..	..	..
131	Australia	17260	2.2	1.6	6	..	..	13	7	9	..	..	..	..
132	Canada	20710	3.3	1.8	4	..	..	5	3	7	..	..	..	..
133	Switzerland	36080	1.5	1.4	4	..	..	13	3	10	49	0	..	..
134	United Kingdom	17790	2.0	2.4	6	..	..	13	3	11	..	..	..	..
135	Austria	22380	4.0	2.0	4	..	..	13	9	2	..	..	..	..
136	Netherlands	20480	2.7	1.7	2	..	..	12	11	5	..	..	..	..
137	Norway	25820	3.6	2.2	5	..	..	10	9	8	..	..	..	..
138	Germany	23030	3.0x	2.4	3	..	..	19x	1x	8x	..	..	..	..
139	Ireland	12210	2.8	3.4	5	..	..	13	12	3	..	..	..	..
140	Hong Kong	15360	6.2	5.5	8	..	..	..	17x	..	37	0	..	..
141	Denmark	26000	2.2	2.1	5	..	..	1x	9x	5x	..	..	..	..
142	Japan	28190	5.1	3.6	2	..	..	..	..	..	..	..	..	..
143	Singapore	15730	8.3	5.3	2	..	..	5	20	24	20	0	1	..
144	Sweden	27010	2.0	1.5	7	..	..	1	9	6	..	..	..	..
145	Finland	21970	3.6	2.0	6	..	..	11	15	5	..	..	..	..

Countries listed in descending order of their 1993 under-five mortality rates (table 1).

Table 7: Women

		Life expectancy females as a % of males 1993	Adult literacy rate females as a % of males 1990	Enrolment ratios females as a % of males 1986-92 primary school	Enrolment ratios females as a % of males 1986-92 secondary school	Contraceptive prevalence (%) 1980-93	% of pregnant women immunized against tetanus 1990-93	% of births attended by trained health personnel 1983-93	Maternal mortality rate 1980-92
1	Niger	107	43	57	44	4	43	15	700
2	Angola	107	52	92	..	1x	14	15	..
3	Sierra Leone	107	35	70	57	4	81	25	450
4	Mozambique	107	47	72	50	4	24	25	300
5	Afghanistan	102	32	53	50	2x	9	9	640
6	Guinea-Bissau	107	48	55	20x	1x	62	27	700x
7	Guinea	102	37	48	36	1x	61	25	800
8	Malawi	105	52x	83	60	13	69	55	400
9	Liberia	106	58	55x	39x	6	20	58	..
10	Mali	107	59	59	44	5	45	32	2000
11	Somalia	107	39	53x	56x	1	5x	2x	1100
12	Chad	107	43	46	20	1x	4	15	960
13	Eritrea	..	..	..	..	..	4	..	..
14	Ethiopia	107	48x	72	71	2	12	14	560x
15	Zambia	105	80	91	56	15	18	51	150
16	Mauritania	106	45	76	53	4	36	40	..
17	Bhutan	102	49	61	29	2	43	7	1310
18	Nigeria	106	65	78	71	6	33	37	800
19	Zaire	106	73	74	47	1x	25	..	800
20	Uganda	105	56	82x	50	5	83	38	550
21	Cambodia	106	46	..	..	..	22	47	500
22	Burundi	109	66	82	40x	9	56	19	..
23	Central African Rep.	109	48	61	41	..	43	66	600
24	Burkina Faso	106	32	63	50x	8	36	42	810
25	Ghana	107	73	82	62	13	6	59	1000
26	Tanzania, U. Rep. of	106	50x	97	67	10	15	53	340x
27	Madagascar	106	83	98	95	17	16	56	570
28	Lesotho	109	..	120	148	23	34	40	..
29	Gabon	106	66	..	..	..	86	80	190
30	Benin	107	50	50	40x	9	77	45	160
31	Lao Peo. Dem. Rep.	106	83x	75	63	..	24	..	300
32	Rwanda	107	58	97	78	21	88	26	210
33	Pakistan	100	45	56	45	12	46	35	500
34	Yemen	100	49	39	21	7	12	16	..
35	Togo	108	55	65	34	12	81	54	420
36	Haiti	107	80	93	95	10	12	20	600
37	Sudan	104	28	77	80	9	9	69	550
38	Nepal	98	34	50	40	23	13	6	830
39	Bangladesh	100	47	86	48	40	80	5	600
40	India	102	55	75	59	43	80	33	460
41	Côte d'Ivoire	106	60	72	50	3	51	50	..
42	Senegal	104	48	72	52	7	30	46	600
43	Bolivia	108	84	91	84	30	52	55	600
44	Cameroon	105	65	85	68	16	49	64	430
45	Indonesia	107	85	96	84	50	67	32	450
46	Myanmar	107	81	93	92	13	66	57	460
47	Congo	110	63	..	..	..	53	..	900
48	Libyan Arab Jamahiriya	105	67	..	..	..	45	76	70x
49	Papua New Guinea	104	58	86	63	4	27	20	900
50	Kenya	107	74	96	70x	33	72	54	170x
51	Turkmenistan	..	98x	..	..	..	..	..	..
52	Turkey	108	79	96	67	63	22	77	150
53	Zimbabwe	106	81	98	78	43	60	70	..
54	Tajikistan	..	98x	..	..	..	..	..	..
55	Namibia	103	..	113	131	29	40	68	370x
56	Mongolia	103	..	104	114x	..	..	99	200
57	Guatemala	108	75	87	85x	23	18	51	200
58	Nicaragua	106	92x	106	144	49	12	73	..
59	Iraq	105	70	85	63	18	44	50	120
60	South Africa	110	96x	..	..	50	26	..	84x
61	Algeria	105	66	85	80	51	36	15	140x
62	Uzbekistan	..	98x	..	..	..	..	..	..
63	Brazil	108	99	96x	116x	66	21	95	200
64	Peru	106	87	96x	91x	59	30	52	300
65	El Salvador	108	92	101	100	53	26	66	..
66	Egypt	103	54	85	81	47	78	41	270
67	Morocco	105	62	69	73	42	80	31	330
68	Philippines	106	99	98	106	40	66	53	100
69	Kyrgyzstan	..	96x	..	..	..	..	..	..
70	Ecuador	106	93	98	104	53	5	84	170
71	Botswana	110	77	104	114	33	46	78	250
72	Honduras	106	93	105	..	47	16	81	220
73	Iran, Islamic Rep. of	101	67	89	74	49	50	70	120
74	Azerbaijan	..	97x	..	..	..	..	..	..
75	Kazakhstan	..	97x	..	..	..	..	..	..

		Life expectancy females as a % of males 1993	Adult literacy rate females as a % of males 1990	Enrolment ratios females as a % of males 1986-92 primary school	Enrolment ratios females as a % of males 1986-92 secondary school	Contraceptive prevalence (%) 1980-93	% of pregnant women immunized against tetanus 1990-93	% of births attended by trained health personnel 1983-93	Maternal mortality rate 1980-92
76	Dominican Rep.	106	96	101	130x	56	24	92	..
77	Viet Nam	106	91	94x	93x	53	71	95	120
78	China	106	78	93	80	83	3	94	95
79	Albania	108	..	101	88	..	..	99	..
80	Lebanon	106	83	96	103	55x	..	45	..
81	Syrian Arab Rep.	106	65	90	77	52	86	61	140
82	Saudi Arabia	104	66	88	80	..	63	90	41
83	Moldova	..	95x	..	..	..	..	..	..
84	Tunisia	103	76	89	82	50	50	69	70
85	Paraguay	108	96	97	103	48	54	66	300
86	Armenia	..	99x	..	..	..	..	..	..
87	Thailand	107	96	96	94	66	86	71	50
88	Mexico	110	94	97	98	53	68	77	110
89	Korea, Dem. Peo. Rep.	109	..	93	..	..	97	100	41
90	Russian Federation	..	98x	..	..	..	..	..	..
91	Romania	109	96	100	99	58x	..	100	72
92	Oman	106	..	92	87	9	95	60	..
93	Georgia	..	99x	..	..	..	..	..	..
94	Jordan	106	79	102	98	35	30	87	48x
95	Argentina	110	100	106	110	74	..	87	140
96	Latvia	113	99x	..	..	..	..	..	..
97	Ukraine	..	98x	..	..	..	..	..	..
98	Venezuela	110	103	102	138	49x	60	69	..
99	Estonia	113	100x	..	..	..	..	..	..
100	Belarus	..	98x	..	..	..	..	..	..
101	Mauritius	110	88	104	108	75	78	85	99
102	Yugoslavia (former)	109	91	100	95x	55x	..	86	27
103	United Arab Emirates	106	66x	97	112	..	..	99	..
104	Trinidad and Tobago	107	97x	100	101	53	..	98	110
105	Uruguay	110	99	98	102x	..	13	96	36
106	Lithuania	115	99x	..	..	..	..	..	..
107	Panama	106	99	96	109	58	27	96	60
108	Bulgaria	109	..	98	104	76x	..	100	9
109	Sri Lanka	106	89	96	108	62	51	94	80
110	Colombia	109	99	102	118	66	40	94	200
111	Slovakia	..	..	..	..	74	..	..	..
112	Chile	110	99	98	107	43x	..	98	35
113	Malaysia	106	81	100	104	48	81	87	59
114	Costa Rica	107	100	99	107	75	68	93	36
115	Poland	113	99x	98	105	75x	..	100	11
116	Hungary	112	99x	100	100	73	..	99	15
117	Jamaica	106	101	103	112	66	50	82	120
118	Kuwait	107	87	98	100	35	44	99	6
119	Portugal	110	91	96	117	66x	..	90	10
120	Cuba	105	98	99	116	70	98	90	39
121	United States	108	..	100	100	74	..	99	8
122	Czech Rep.	..	..	..	..	78	..	..	..
123	Greece	107	91	101	98	..	..	97	5
124	Belgium	108	..	102	101	79	..	100	3
125	Spain	108	96	99	109	59	..	96	5
126	France	111	..	98	105	80	..	94	9
127	Korea, Rep. of	109	94	103	101	79	..	89	26
128	Israel	104	94x	103	109	..	..	99	3
129	Italy	108	98	100	100	78x	..	..	4
130	New Zealand	108	..	99	101	70x	..	99	13
131	Australia	108	..	100	102	76	..	99	3
132	Canada	109	..	98	100	73	..	99	5
133	Switzerland	108	..	101	94	71	..	99	5
134	United Kingdom	107	..	101	104	72	..	100	8
135	Austria	108	..	99	94	71	..	..	8
136	Netherlands	109	..	103	97	76	..	100	10
137	Norway	109	..	100	101	76	..	..	3
138	Germany	108	..	100	97	75	..	99	5
139	Ireland	107	..	100	109	..	..	..	2
140	Hong Kong	107	71x	100	103x	81	..	100	6
141	Denmark	108	..	100	103	78	..	100	3
142	Japan	108	..	..	102	64	..	100	11
143	Singapore	107	80x	97	101	74	..	100	10
144	Sweden	108	..	100	104	78	..	100	5
145	Finland	111	..	100	119	80x	..	100	11

Countries listed in descending order of their 1993 under-five mortality rates (table 1).

Table 8: Basic indicators on less populous countries

		Under-5 mortality rate 1960	Under-5 mortality rate 1993	Infant mortality rate (under 1) 1960	Infant mortality rate (under 1) 1993	Total population (thousands) 1993	Annual no. of births (thousands) 1993	Annual no. of under-5 deaths (thousands) 1993	GNP per capita (US$) 1992	Life expectancy at birth (years) 1993	Total adult literacy rate 1985-90	% of age group enrolled in primary school (gross) 1986-92	% of children immunized against measles 1991-93
1	Gambia	375	216	213	131	932	40.7	8.8	370	45	27	68	87
2	Equatorial Guinea	316	180	188	116	379	16.5	3.0	330	48	62x	149x	53
3	Djibouti	289	158	186	113	481	22.4	3.5	1210x	49	12	39	42
4	Comoros	248	128	165	88	607	29.5	3.8	510	56	48x	75	56
5	Swaziland	233	107	157	74	814	30.3	3.3	1090	58	67	111	85
6	Marshall Islands	..	92	..	63	51	1.6x	0.1	*	..	91	95	86
7	Sao Tome/Principe	..	84	..	64	127	4.6	0.4	360	68	57x	..	57
8	Vanuatu	..	84	..	64	161	6.1	0.5	1210	65	64	103	66
9	Kiribati	..	80	..	59	75	2.5	0.2	700	56	93	91	77
10	Maldives	258	78	158	56	234	9.0	0.7	500	64	91	25	86
11	Cape Verde	164	73	110	54	395	14.0	1.0	850	68	66	115	95
12	Guyana	126	63	100	47	816	20.4	1.3	330	65	96	112	80
13	Samoa	..	57	..	44	158	5.2	0.3	940	66	98	100	81
14	Tuvalu	..	56	..	40	13	..	..	650x	..	99	101	88
15	Belize	104	42	74	33	202	7.5	0.3	2220	69	93	90	80
16	Saint Kitts/Nevis	..	41	..	33	42	0.8	0.0	3990	71	90	..	99
17	Palau	..	35	..	25	16	0.3x	0.0	790x	..	98	103	92
18	Grenada	..	35	..	28	92	2.3	0.1	2310	71	98x	88x	99
19	Suriname	96	34	70	28	446	11.3	0.4	4280	70	95	127	61
20	Solomon Islands	185	33	120	27	354	13.2	0.4	710	71	62	104	64
21	British Virgin Islands	..	31	..	26	18	0.4x	0.0	8500x	..	98x	..	99
22	Turks/Caicos Islands	..	31	..	25	13	0.3x	0.0	780x	..	98x	..	59
23	Micronesia, Fed. States of	..	29	..	24	114	3.9	0.1	*	71	81	100	88
24	Bahamas	68	29	51	24	268	5.2	0.2	12070	72	..	99	93
25	Cook Islands	..	28	..	26	17	0.4x	0.0	1550x	..	99	98	87
26	Fiji	97	28	71	23	747	17.4	0.5	2010	72	87	126	96
27	Tonga	..	25	..	21	98	2.9	0.1	1480	68	99	98	90
28	Qatar	239	25	145	20	466	10.4	0.3	16750	70	76	99	86
29	Antigua/Barbuda	..	24	..	20	67	1.1	0.0	5980	74	95	100	99
30	Saint Vincent/Grenadines	..	24	..	20	110	2.4	0.1	1990	71	82	95x	99
31	Saint Lucia	..	22	..	18	139	3.9	0.1	2920	72	82x	95x	94
32	Bahrain	208	22	130	18	548	14.2	0.3	7130x	71	77	95	90
33	Dominica	..	22	..	18	72	1.6	0.0	2520	73	94x	..	99
34	Seychelles	..	20	..	16	72	1.7	0.0	5460	71	88	102x	92
35	Montserrat	..	15	..	12	11	0.2	0.0	3330x	74	97x	100x	99
36	Malta	42	12	37	10	361	5.5	0.1	7280x	76	86	110	92
37	Cyprus	36	10	30	9	723	12.1	0.1	9820	77	94	103	83
38	Barbados	90	10	74	9	260	4.1	0.0	6540	76	98	106	92
39	Luxembourg	41	10	33	9	380	4.7	0.0	35160	76	..	90	80
40	Brunei Darussalam	87	10	63	8	276	6.5	0.1	20760x	74	78x	110	92
41	Iceland	22	6	17	5	263	4.6	0.0	23880	78	..	101	98

* Range $676-$2695.

MEASURING HUMAN DEVELOPMENT
An introduction to table 9

If development in the 1990s is to assume a more human face then there arises a corresponding need for a means of measuring human as well as economic progress. From UNICEF's point of view, in particular, there is a need for an agreed method of measuring the level of child well-being and its rate of change.

The under-five mortality rate (U5MR) is used in table 9 (next page) as the principal indicator of such progress.

The U5MR has several advantages. First, it measures an end result of the development process rather than an 'input' such as school enrolment level, per capita calorie availability, or the number of doctors per thousand population – all of which are means to an end.

Second, the U5MR is known to be the result of a wide variety of inputs: the nutritional health and the health knowledge of mothers; the level of immunization and ORT use; the availability of maternal and child health services (including prenatal care); income and food availability in the family; the availability of clean water and safe sanitation; and the overall safety of the child's environment.

Third, the U5MR is less susceptible than, say, per capita GNP to the fallacy of the average. This is because the natural scale does not allow the children of the rich to be one thousand times as likely to survive, even if the man-made scale does permit them to have one thousand times as much income. In other words, it is much more difficult for a wealthy minority to affect a nation's U5MR, and it therefore presents a more accurate, if far from perfect, picture of the health status of the majority of children (and of society as a whole).

For these reasons, the U5MR is chosen by UNICEF as its single most important indicator of the state of a nation's children. That is why the statistical annex lists the nations of the world not in ascending order of their per capita GNP but in descending order of their under-five mortality rates.

The speed of progress in reducing the U5MR can be measured by calculating its average annual reduction rate (AARR). Unlike the comparison of absolute changes, the AARR reflects the fact that the lower limits to U5MR are approached only with increasing difficulty. As lower levels of under-five mortality are reached, for example, the same absolute reduction obviously represents a greater percentage of reduction. The AARR therefore shows a higher rate of progress for, say, a 10 point reduction if that reduction happens at a lower level of under-five mortality. (A fall in U5MR of 10 points from 100 to 90 represents a reduction of 10%, whereas the same 10-point fall from 20 to 10 represents a reduction of 50%.)

When used in conjunction with GNP growth rates, the U5MR and its reduction rate can therefore give a picture of the progress being made by any country or region, and over any period of time, towards the satisfaction of some of the most essential of human needs.

As table 9 shows, there is no fixed relationship between the annual reduction rate of the U5MR and the annual rate of growth in per capita GNP. Such comparisons help to throw the emphasis on to the policies, priorities, and other factors which determine the ratio between economic and social progress.

Finally, the table gives the total fertility rate for each country and its average annual rate of reduction. It will be seen that many of the nations which have achieved significant reductions in their U5MR have also achieved significant reductions in fertility.

Table 9: The rate of progress

		Under-5 mortality rate			average annual rate of reduction (%)			GNP per capita average annual growth rate (%)		Total fertility rate			average annual rate of reduction (%)	
		1960	1980	1993	1960-80	1980-93	required* 1993-2000	1965-80	1980-92	1960	1980	1993	1960-80	1980-93
1	Niger	320	320	320	0.0	0.0	21.7	-2.5	-4.3	7.1	7.1	7.1	0.0	0.0
2	Angola	345	261	292	1.4	-0.9	20.4	..	6.1x	6.4	6.9	7.1	-0.4	-0.2
3	Sierra Leone	385	301	284	1.2	0.4	20.0	0.7	-1.4	6.2	6.5	6.5	-0.2	0.0
4	Mozambique	331	269	282	1.0	-0.4	19.9	..	-3.6	6.3	6.5	6.5	-0.2	0.0
5	Afghanistan	360	280	257	1.3	0.7	18.6	0.6	..	6.9	7.1	6.8	-0.1	0.3
6	Guinea-Bissau	336	290	235	0.7	1.6	17.3	-2.7	1.6	5.1	5.7	5.8	-0.6	-0.1
7	Guinea	337	276	226	1.0	1.5	16.8	1.3	..	7.0	7.0	7.0	0.0	0.0
8	Malawi	365	290	223	1.1	2.0	16.6	3.2	-0.1	6.9	7.6	7.5	-0.5	0.1
9	Liberia	288	235	217	1.0	0.6	16.2	0.5	5.2x	6.6	6.8	6.8	-0.1	0.0
10	Mali	400	310	217	1.3	2.7	16.2	2.1x	-2.7	7.1	7.1	7.1	0.0	0.0
11	Somalia	294	246	211	0.9	1.2	15.8	-0.1	-1.8x	7.0	7.0	7.0	0.0	0.0
12	Chad	325	254	206	1.2	1.6	15.4	-1.9	3.4	6.0	5.9	5.9	0.1	0.0
13	Eritrea	294	260	204	0.6	1.9	15.3	..	..	..	..	5.8	..	..
14	Ethiopia	294	260	204	0.6	1.9	15.3	0.4	-1.9	6.7	6.8	7.0	-0.1	-0.2
15	Zambia	220	160	203	1.6	-1.8	15.2	-1.2	-2.9x	6.6	7.1	6.3	-0.4	0.9
16	Mauritania	321	249	202	1.3	1.6	15.2	-0.1	-0.8	6.5	6.5	6.5	0.0	0.0
17	Bhutan	324	249	197	1.3	1.8	14.8	..	6.3	6.0	5.9	5.8	0.1	0.1
18	Nigeria	204	196	191	0.2	0.2	14.3	4.2	-0.4	6.8	6.9	6.4	-0.1	0.6
19	Zaire	286	204	187	1.7	0.7	14.0	-1.3	-1.6x	6.0	6.6	6.7	-0.5	-0.1
20	Uganda	218	181	185	0.9	-0.2	13.9	-2.2	3.3x	6.9	7.0	7.2	-0.1	-0.2
21	Cambodia	217	330	181	-2.1	4.6	13.5	..	..	6.3	4.5	4.5	1.7	0.0
22	Burundi	255	193	178	1.4	0.6	13.3	2.4	1.3	6.8	6.8	6.7	0.0	0.1
23	Central African Rep.	294	202	177	1.9	1.0	13.2	0.8	-1.5	5.6	6.0	6.2	-0.3	-0.3
24	Burkina Faso	318	246	175	1.3	2.6	13.1	1.7	1.0	6.4	6.5	6.5	-0.1	0.0
25	Ghana	215	157	170	1.6	-0.6	12.7	-0.8	-0.1	6.9	6.5	5.9	0.3	0.7
26	Tanzania, U. Rep. of	249	202	167	1.0	1.5	12.5	0.8	0.0	6.8	6.8	6.8	0.0	0.0
27	Madagascar	364	216	164	2.6	2.1	12.2	-0.4	-2.4	6.6	6.6	6.6	0.0	0.0
28	Lesotho	204	173	156	0.8	0.8	11.4	6.8	-0.5	5.8	5.6	4.7	0.2	1.3
29	Gabon	287	194	154	2.0	1.8	11.3	5.6	-3.7	4.1	4.4	5.4	-0.4	-1.6
30	Benin	310	176	144	2.8	1.5	10.3	-0.3	-0.7	6.9	7.1	7.1	-0.1	0.0
31	Lao Peo. Dem. Rep.	233	190	141	1.0	2.3	10.0	..	1.2x	6.2	6.7	6.6	-0.4	0.1
32	Rwanda	191	222	141	-0.8	3.5	10.0	1.6	-0.6	7.5	8.5	8.4	-0.6	0.1
33	Pakistan	221	151	137	1.9	0.7	9.6	1.8	3.1	6.9	7.0	6.1	-0.1	1.1
34	Yemen	378	210	137	2.9	3.3	9.6	..	..	7.5	7.7	7.1	-0.1	0.6
35	Togo	264	175	135	2.0	2.0	9.4	1.7	-1.8	6.6	6.6	6.5	0.0	0.1
36	Haiti	270	195	130	1.6	3.1	8.9	0.9	-2.4x	6.3	5.3	4.8	0.9	0.8
37	Sudan	292	200	128	1.9	3.4	8.7	0.8	-2.4x	6.7	6.6	6.0	0.1	0.7
38	Nepal	279	177	128	2.3	2.5	8.6	..	2.0	5.8	6.4	5.4	-0.5	1.3
39	Bangladesh	247	211	122	0.8	4.2	7.9	-0.3	1.8	6.7	6.4	4.7	0.2	2.4
40	India	236	177	122	1.4	2.9	7.9	1.5	3.1	5.9	4.8	3.8	1.0	1.8
41	Côte d'Ivoire	300	180	120	2.6	3.1	7.7	2.8	-4.7	7.2	7.4	7.4	-0.1	0.0
42	Senegal	303	221	120	1.6	4.7	7.7	-0.5	0.1	7.0	6.9	6.0	0.1	1.1
43	Bolivia	252	170	114	2.0	3.1	7.0	1.7	-1.5	6.7	5.8	4.5	0.7	2.0
44	Cameroon	264	173	113	2.1	3.3	6.9	2.4	-1.5	5.8	6.4	5.7	-0.5	0.9
45	Indonesia	216	128	111	2.6	1.1	6.6	5.2	4.0	5.5	4.4	3.1	1.1	2.7
46	Myanmar	237	146	111	2.4	2.1	6.6	1.6	..	6.0	5.1	4.1	0.8	1.7
47	Congo	220	125	109	2.8	1.0	6.4	2.7	-0.8	5.9	6.3	6.2	-0.3	0.1
48	Libyan Arab Jamahiriya	269	150	100	2.9	3.1	5.0	0.0	-9.2x	7.1	7.3	6.3	-0.1	1.1
49	Papua New Guinea	248	95	95	4.8	0.0	5.8	..	0.0	6.3	5.7	4.8	0.5	1.3
50	Kenya	202	112	90	2.9	1.7	5.8	3.1	0.2	8.0	7.8	6.2	0.1	1.8
51	Turkmenistan	..	..	89	..	..	..	..	0.7x	..	..	4.5	..	..
52	Turkey	217	141	84	2.2	4.0	4.1	3.6	2.9	6.3	4.3	3.4	1.9	1.8
53	Zimbabwe	181	125	83	1.8	3.1	4.6	1.7	-0.9	7.5	6.4	5.3	0.8	1.5
54	Tajikistan	..	..	83	..	..	..	..	-0.1x	..	..	5.3	..	..
55	Namibia	206	114	79	3.0	2.9	4.9	..	-1.0	6.0	6.0	6.0	0.0	0.0
56	Mongolia	185	112	78	2.5	2.8	4.7	..	..	6.0	5.4	4.6	0.5	1.2
57	Guatemala	205	136	73	2.0	4.8	3.7	3.0	-1.5	6.9	6.3	5.3	0.5	1.3
58	Nicaragua	209	143	72	1.9	5.3	3.2	-0.7	-5.3	7.4	6.2	5.0	0.9	1.7
59	Iraq	171	83	71	3.6	1.2	11.4	..	..	7.2	6.5	5.7	0.5	1.0
60	South Africa	126	91	69	1.6	2.1	5.0	3.2	0.1	6.5	4.9	4.1	1.4	1.4
61	Algeria	243	145	68	2.6	5.8	3.7	4.2	-0.5	7.3	6.8	4.8	0.4	2.7
62	Uzbekistan	..	..	66	..	..	..	..	0.8x	..	..	4.3	..	..
63	Brazil	181	93	63	3.3	3.0	4.5	6.3	0.4	6.2	4.0	2.7	2.2	3.0
64	Peru	236	130	62	3.0	5.8	3.2	0.8	-2.8	6.9	5.0	3.5	1.6	2.7
65	El Salvador	210	120	60	2.8	5.4	3.5	1.5	0.0	6.8	5.4	4.0	1.2	2.3
66	Egypt	258	180	59	1.8	8.6	1.5	2.8	1.8	7.0	5.2	4.1	1.5	1.8
67	Morocco	215	145	59	2.0	6.9	2.9	2.7	1.4	7.2	5.7	4.3	1.2	2.2
68	Philippines	102	70	59	1.9	1.3	5.0	3.2	-1.0	6.9	4.9	3.9	1.7	1.8
69	Kyrgyzstan	..	..	58	..	..	..	..	2.1x	..	..	3.9	..	..
70	Ecuador	180	101	57	2.9	4.4	4.3	5.4	-0.3	6.9	5.1	3.6	1.5	2.7
71	Botswana	170	94	56	3.0	4.0	4.4	9.9	6.1	6.8	6.8	5.0	0.0	2.4
72	Honduras	203	100	56	3.6	4.4	4.3	1.1	-0.3	7.3	6.4	4.9	0.7	2.1
73	Iran, Islamic Rep. of	233	126	54	3.1	6.5	2.8	2.9	-1.4	7.2	6.5	5.9	0.5	0.7
74	Azerbaijan	..	..	52	..	..	..	..	0.4x	..	..	3.2	..	..
75	Kazakhstan	..	..	49	..	..	..	..	0.9x	..	..	2.7	..	..

		Under-5 mortality rate						GNP per capita average annual growth rate (%)		Total fertility rate				
					average annual rate of reduction (%)								average annual rate of reduction (%)	
		1960	1980	1993	1960-80	1980-93	required* 1993-2000	1965-80	1980-92	1960	1980	1993	1960-80	1980-93
76	Dominican Rep.	152	94	48	2.4	5.2	3.5	3.8	-0.5	7.4	4.5	3.3	2.5	2.4
77	Viet Nam	219	105	48	3.7	6.1	3.8	..	..	6.0	5.1	3.8	0.8	2.3
78	China	209	65	43	5.9	3.1	5.8	4.1	7.6	5.7	2.7	2.2	3.7	1.6
79	Albania	151	57	41	4.9	2.6	5.8	..	..	5.9	3.8	2.7	2.2	2.6
80	Lebanon	85	40	40	3.8	0.0	5.8	..	..	6.3	4.0	3.1	2.3	2.0
81	Syrian Arab Rep.	201	73	39	5.1	4.8	4.0	5.1	-1.4x	7.3	7.4	6.1	-0.1	1.5
82	Saudi Arabia	292	90	38	5.9	6.6	3.4	4.0x	-3.3	7.2	7.3	6.3	-0.1	1.1
83	Moldova	..	..	36	..	..	..	..	1.8x	..	..	2.5	..	..
84	Tunisia	244	102	36	4.4	8.0	2.3	4.7	1.3	7.1	5.3	3.4	1.5	3.4
85	Paraguay	90	61	34	1.9	4.5	4.6	4.1	-0.7	6.8	4.9	4.3	1.6	1.0
86	Armenia	..	..	33	..	..	..	..	2.1x	..	..	3.0	..	..
87	Thailand	146	61	33	4.4	4.7	4.2	4.4	6.0	6.4	3.6	2.2	2.9	3.8
88	Mexico	141	81	32	2.8	7.0	3.2	3.6	-0.2	6.8	4.7	3.1	1.8	3.2
89	Korea, Dem. Peo. Rep.	120	43	32	5.1	2.4	4.5	..	..	5.8	3.1	2.4	3.1	2.0
90	Russian Federation	..	..	31	..	..	..	..	1.3x	..	..	1.8	..	..
91	Romania	82	36	29	4.1	1.6	3.9	..	-1.1	2.3	2.4	2.1	-0.2	1.0
92	Oman	300	95	29	5.7	9.2	3.1	9.0	4.1	7.2	7.2	6.7	0.0	0.6
93	Georgia	..	..	28	..	..	..	..	2.2x	..	..	2.1	..	..
94	Jordan	149	66	27	4.1	6.7	2.4	5.8x	-5.4	7.7	7.1	5.7	0.4	1.7
95	Argentina	68	41	27	2.5	3.3	5.8	1.7	-0.9	3.1	3.3	2.8	-0.3	1.3
96	Latvia	..	..	26	..	..	..	..	0.2	1.9	2.0	2.0	-0.3	0.0
97	Ukraine	..	..	25	..	..	..	..	2.3x	..	..	1.8	..	..
98	Venezuela	70	42	24	2.6	4.3	4.6	2.3	-0.8	6.5	4.2	3.1	2.2	2.3
99	Estonia	..	..	23	..	..	..	..	-2.3	2.0	2.1	2.1	-0.2	0.0
100	Belarus	..	..	22	..	..	..	..	3.3x	..	..	1.9	..	..
101	Mauritius	84	42	22	3.4	5.0	3.6	3.7	5.6	5.9	2.8	2.0	3.7	2.6
102	Yugoslavia (former)	113	37	22	5.6	4.0	5.2	5.2	-1.4x	2.8	2.1	1.9	1.4	0.8
103	United Arab Emirates	240	64	21	6.6	8.5	4.0	..	-4.3	6.9	5.4	4.5	1.2	1.4
104	Trinidad and Tobago	73	40	21	3.0	5.0	3.7	3.1	-2.6	5.2	3.3	2.7	2.3	1.5
105	Uruguay	47	42	21	0.6	5.3	4.2	2.5	-1.0	2.9	2.7	2.3	0.4	1.2
106	Lithuania	..	..	20	..	..	..	..	-1.0	2.5	2.1	2.0	0.9	0.4
107	Panama	104	31	20	6.0	3.4	5.2	2.8	-1.2	5.9	3.8	2.8	2.2	2.3
108	Bulgaria	70	25	19	5.1	1.9	6.9	..	1.2	2.2	2.1	1.8	0.2	1.2
109	Sri Lanka	130	52	19	4.6	7.7	3.1	2.8	2.6	5.3	3.5	2.5	2.1	2.6
110	Colombia	132	59	19	4.1	8.7	4.2	3.7	1.4	6.8	3.8	2.6	2.9	2.9
111	Slovakia	..	..	18	..	..	..	..	..	..	..	2.0	..	..
112	Chile	138	35	17	6.9	5.5	3.4	0.0	3.7	5.3	2.8	2.7	3.2	0.3
113	Malaysia	105	42	17	4.6	6.9	3.0	4.7	3.2	6.8	4.2	3.6	2.4	1.2
114	Costa Rica	112	29	16	6.8	4.5	5.7	3.3	0.8	7.0	3.7	3.1	3.2	1.4
115	Poland	70	24	15	5.3	3.6	3.4	..	0.1	3.0	2.3	2.1	1.3	0.7
116	Hungary	57	26	15	3.9	4.4	4.2	5.1	0.2	2.0	2.0	1.8	0.0	0.8
117	Jamaica	76	39	13	3.4	8.2	3.2	-0.1	0.2	5.4	3.8	2.3	1.8	3.9
118	Kuwait	128	35	13	6.6	7.6	2.4	0.6x	-2.2x	7.3	5.4	3.7	1.5	2.9
119	Portugal	112	31	11	6.4	7.7	0.8	4.6	3.1	3.1	2.2	1.5	1.7	2.9
120	Cuba	50	26	10	3.3	7.0	2.6	..	..	4.2	2.0	1.9	3.7	0.4
121	United States	30	15	10	3.3	3.1	4.8	1.8	1.7	3.5	1.8	2.1	3.3	-1.2
122	Czech Rep.	..	..	10	..	..	..	..	..	..	..	1.9	..	..
123	Greece	64	23	10	5.2	6.7	3.7	4.8	1.0	2.2	2.1	1.5	0.2	2.6
124	Belgium	35	15	10	4.3	3.4	5.9	3.6	2.0	2.6	1.7	1.7	2.1	0.0
125	Spain	57	16	9	6.2	4.3	5.6	4.1	2.9	2.8	2.2	1.4	1.2	3.5
126	France	34	13	9	4.9	2.7	5.4	3.7	1.7	2.8	1.9	1.8	1.9	0.4
127	Korea, Rep. of	124	18	9	9.8	5.2	3.6	7.3	8.5	5.7	2.6	1.8	3.9	2.8
128	Israel	39	19	9	3.6	6.1	1.6	3.7	1.9	3.9	3.3	2.8	0.8	1.3
129	Italy	50	17	9	5.3	5.3	4.0	3.2	2.2	2.4	1.7	1.3	1.7	2.1
130	New Zealand	26	16	9	2.5	4.6	0.5	1.7	0.6	3.9	2.1	2.1	3.1	0.0
131	Australia	24	13	8	3.0	3.6	4.1	2.2	1.6	3.3	2.0	1.9	2.5	0.4
132	Canada	33	13	8	4.8	3.4	5.2	3.3	1.8	3.8	1.7	1.8	4.0	-0.4
133	Switzerland	27	11	8	4.5	2.6	3.5	1.5	1.4	2.4	1.5	1.7	2.4	-1.0
134	United Kingdom	27	14	8	3.1	4.6	3.5	2.0	2.4	2.7	1.8	1.9	2.0	-0.4
135	Austria	43	17	8	4.6	6.1	2.9	4.0	2.0	2.7	1.6	1.5	2.6	0.5
136	Netherlands	22	11	8	3.4	2.8	4.1	2.7	1.7	3.1	1.5	1.7	3.6	-1.0
137	Norway	23	11	8	3.8	2.6	2.5	3.6	2.2	2.9	1.7	2.0	2.7	-1.3
138	Germany	40	16	7	4.7	5.8	3.2	3.0x	2.8	2.4	1.5	1.5	2.4	0.0
139	Ireland	36	14	7	4.6	5.3	2.6	2.8	3.4	3.8	3.2	2.1	0.9	3.2
140	Hong Kong	52	13	7	6.9	4.8	5.1	6.2	5.5	5.0	2.1	1.5	4.3	2.6
141	Denmark	25	10	7	4.4	3.2	1.8	2.2	2.1	2.6	1.6	1.7	2.4	-0.5
142	Japan	40	11	6	6.6	3.9	6.1	5.1	3.6	2.0	1.8	1.7	0.5	0.4
143	Singapore	40	13	6	5.6	6.2	1.3	8.3	5.3	5.5	1.8	1.8	5.6	0.0
144	Sweden	20	9	6	4.1	3.3	3.4	2.0	1.5	2.3	1.6	2.1	1.8	-2.1
145	Finland	28	9	5	5.9	4.1	1.8	3.6	2.0	2.7	1.7	1.8	2.3	-0.4

* The average annual reduction rate required to achieve an under-five mortality rate in all countries of 70 per 1000 live births or of two thirds the 1990 rate, whichever is the less. Countries listed in descending order of their 1993 under-five mortality rates.

83

Table 10: Regional summaries

	Sub-Saharan Africa	Middle East and North Africa	South Asia	East Asia and Pacific	Latin America and Caribbean	Former USSR	Industrialized countries	Developing countries	Least developed countries
Table 1: Basic indicators									
Under-5 mortality rate 1960	255	240	238	200	157	..	43	216	282
Under-5 mortality rate 1993	179	70	127	56	48	42	10	102	173
Infant mortality rate 1960	152	155	146	132	105	..	36	137	171
Infant mortality rate 1993	109	53	87	42	38	35	9	69	111
Total population (millions)	547	350	1208	1754	459	293	941	4318	550
Annual no. of births (thousands)	24974	12250	38241	39440	11706	4524	12726	126611	24306
Annual no. of under-5 deaths (thousands)	4475	863	4848	2202	565	189	130	12953	4207
GNP per capita (US$)	504	1977	313	800	2648	2015	19521	918	236
Life expectancy at birth (years)	51	64	59	68	68	69	76	62	50
Total adult literacy rate (%)	50	58	46	80	85	99	96	67	43
% enrolled in primary school	67	96	88	117	106	..	102	98	65
% share of household income, lowest 40%	..	..	21	18	10	..	18	..	..
% share of household income, highest 20%	..	..	41	44	62	..	41	..	..
Table 2: Nutrition									
% with low birth weight	16	10	34	11	11	..	6	19	24
% of children who are exclusively breastfed, 0-3 months	26	..	..	..	..	..	..	..	..
% of children who are breastfed with food, 6-9 months	68	..	..	..	..	..	..	..	..
% of children who are still breastfeeding, 20-23 months	..	..	..	..	..	..	..	..	..
% of children suffering from underweight, moderate & severe	31	13	64	27	11	..	..	37	41
% of children suffering from underweight, severe	9	..	24	..	2	..	..	12	..
% of children suffering from wasting, moderate & severe	7	6	12	..	3	..	..	6	10
% of children suffering from stunting, moderate & severe	42	25	63	..	21	..	..	43	51
Total goitre rate (%)	16	23	13	13	15	..	..	15	20
Calorie supply as % of requirements	93	124	99	112	114	..	134	107	90
% share of household consumption, all foods	38	39	51	45	34	..	14	41	..
% share of household consumption, cereals	15	10	19	..	8	..	2	..	..
Table 3: Health									
% with access to safe water, total	42	77	77	66	80	..	..	69	49
% with access to safe water, urban	73	93	84	91	90	..	..	88	64
% with access to safe water, rural	35	61	74	57	55	..	..	60	46
% with access to adequate sanitation, total	36	70	29	27	66	..	..	36	34
% with access to adequate sanitation, urban	58	94	61	63	79	..	..	69	62
% with access to adequate sanitation, rural	28	47	14	13	33	..	..	18	27
% with access to health services, total	56	82	77	87	74	..	..	79	48
% with access to health services, urban	..	..	..	..	..	..	..	..	..
% with access to health services, rural	..	..	..	..	..	..	..	..	..
% of 1-year-olds immunized against TB	62	84	90	92	92	88	77	85	72
% of 1-year-olds immunized against DPT	48	83	84	92	81	70	87	79	55
% of 1-year-olds immunized against polio	48	83	84	92	80	72	92	79	55
% of 1-year-olds immunized against measles	49	80	78	91	85	87	80	78	54
% of pregnant women immunized against tetanus	35	48	70	26	38	..	..	44	41
ORT use rate (%)	49	56	39	36	64	..	..	44	44
Table 4: Education									
Adult literacy rate 1970, male (%)	34	47	44	76	76	..	97	53	36
Adult literacy rate 1970, female (%)	17	19	19	56	69	..	95	33	18
Adult literacy rate 1990, male (%)	61	69	59	88	86	99	..	76	54
Adult literacy rate 1990, female (%)	40	45	32	71	83	97	..	57	32
No. of radio sets per 1000 population	143	238	78	196	345	..	1144	176	95
No. of television sets per 1000 population	23	110	29	44	162	..	551	55	9
Primary school enrolment ratio (%) 1960 (gross), male	47	72	77	120	75	..	109	93	48
Primary school enrolment ratio (%) 1960 (gross), female	24	40	39	85	71	..	107	62	23
Primary school enrolment ratio (%) 1986-92 (gross), male	74	104	101	121	105	..	102	105	73
Primary school enrolment ratio (%) 1986-92 (gross), female	60	89	75	113	103	..	102	90	57
Primary school enrolment ratio (%) 1986-92 (net), male	55	91	..	..	82	..	96	87	56
Primary school enrolment ratio (%) 1986-92 (net), female	46	81	..	..	82	..	97	80	46
% school entrants reaching grade 5, primary school	61	90	59	86	60	..	98	71	54
Secondary school enrolment ratio, male (%)	22	60	47	54	45	..	91	48	21
Secondary school enrolment ratio, female (%)	14	45	28	46	49	..	92	37	12

	Sub-Saharan Africa	Middle East and North Africa	South Asia	East Asia and Pacific	Latin America and Caribbean	Former USSR	Industrialized countries	Developing countries	Least developed countries
Table 5: Demographic indicators									
Population under 16 (millions)	264	153	472	548	169	80	198	1605	255
Population under 5 (millions)	102	55	163	187	55	24	62	561	97
Population annual growth rate 1965-80 (%)	2.8	2.8	2.3	2.2	2.5	..	0.8	2.4	2.6
Population annual growth rate 1980-93 (%)	3.0	2.9	2.2	1.7	2.1	..	0.6	2.1	2.7
Crude death rate 1960	24	21	21	19	13	..	10	20	25
Crude death rate 1993	15	8	11	7	7	11	10	9	15
Crude birth rate 1960	49	47	44	39	42	..	20	42	48
Crude birth rate 1993	45	35	32	23	26	16	13	29	44
Life expectancy 1960 (years)	40	47	43	47	56	..	69	46	39
Life expectancy 1993 (years)	51	64	59	68	68	69	76	62	50
Total fertility rate	6.4	4.9	4.2	2.5	3.0	2.0	1.8	3.6	5.9
% of population urbanized	31	55	26	31	73	66	76	36	22
Urban population annual growth rate 1965-80 (%)	5.4	4.6	3.8	3.3	3.8	..	1.4	3.9	5.5
Urban population annual growth rate 1980-93 (%)	5.1	4.5	3.5	4.1	3.0	..	0.9	3.9	5.2
Table 6: Economic indicators									
GNP per capita (US$)	504	1977	313	800	2648	2015	19521	918	236
GNP per capita annual growth rate 1965-80 (%)	3.0	3.2	1.5	4.8	4.1	..	2.9	3.7	0.4
GNP per capita annual growth rate 1980-92 (%)	-0.4	-0.7	3.0	6.5	0.0	1.5	2.2	2.4	0.3
Annual rate of inflation (%)	15	15	9	7	228	..	5.0	75	16
% below absolute poverty level, urban	..	..	33	..	18	..	..	27	55
% below absolute poverty level, rural	62	..	39	17	49	..	..	31	70
% of government expenditure to health	4	5	2	3	6	..	13	4	5
% of government expenditure to education	12	18	3	16	9	..	4.0	11	13
% of government expenditure to defence	9	15	18	13	5	..	13	11	13
ODA inflow (US$ millions)	16881	7676	6694	9579	4551	..	..	45381	15295
ODA inflow as % of recipient GNP	12	1	2	1	0	..	..	1	18
Debt service, % of goods & services exports 1970	5	..	21	..	14	..	..	12	7
Debt service, % of goods & services exports 1992	16	22	18	9	22	..	..	15	10
Table 7: Women									
Life expectancy, females as % of males	107	104	101	106	108	..	108	105	104
Adult literacy, females as % of males	67	66	54	81	97	99	..	75	58
Enrolment, females as % of males, primary school	81	85	75	94	98	..	100	87	78
Enrolment, females as % of males, secondary school	64	74	58	84	108	..	102	77	56
Contraceptive prevalence (%)	12	44	39	74	59	..	72	54	16
Pregnant women immunized against tetanus (%)	35	48	70	26	38	..	..	44	41
% of births attended by trained health personnel	38	57	29	81	82	..	98	55	27
Maternal mortality rate	616	202	492	159	189	..	10	351	607
Table 9: The rate of progress									
Under-5 mortality rate 1960	255	240	237	200	157	..	43	216	282
Under-5 mortality rate 1980	203	142	179	80	86	..	17	138	221
Under-5 mortality rate 1993	179	71	127	56	48	41	10	102	173
Under-5 mortality annual reduction rate 1960-80 (%)	1.1	2.6	1.4	4.6	3.0	..	4.6	2.2	1.2
Under-5 mortality annual reduction rate 1980-93 (%)	1.0	5.4	2.7	2.8	4.5	..	3.8	2.3	1.9
Under-5 mortality annual reduction rate required 1993-2000 (%)	13.8	5.0	8.6	5.8	4.4	..	4.4	8.8	13.0
GNP per capita annual growth rate 1965-80 (%)	3.0	3.2	1.5	4.8	4.1	..	2.9	3.7	0.4
GNP per capita annual growth rate 1980-92 (%)	-0.4	-0.7	3.0	6.5	0.0	1.5	2.2	2.4	0.3
Total fertility rate 1960	6.7	7.0	6.1	5.8	6.0	..	2.8	6.1	6.6
Total fertility rate 1980	6.7	5.9	5.2	3.2	4.2	..	1.9	4.4	6.5
Total fertility rate 1993	6.4	4.9	4.2	2.5	3.0	2.0	1.8	3.6	5.9
Total fertility annual reduction rate 1960-80 (%)	0.0	0.9	0.8	3.0	1.8	..	2.0	1.6	0.0
Total fertility annual reduction rate 1980-93 (%)	0.3	1.4	1.7	1.8	2.5	..	0.1	1.5	0.7

Figures in this table are totals or weighted averages.

COUNTRY GROUPINGS

SUB-SAHARAN AFRICA

Angola	Eritrea	Malawi	Sierra Leone
Benin	Ethiopia	Mali	Somalia
Botswana	Gabon	Mauritania	South Africa
Burkina Faso	Ghana	Mauritius	Tanzania, U. Rep. of
Burundi	Guinea	Mozambique	Togo
Cameroon	Guinea-Bissau	Namibia	Uganda
Central African Rep.	Kenya	Niger	Zaire
Chad	Lesotho	Nigeria	Zambia
Congo	Liberia	Rwanda	Zimbabwe
Côte d'Ivoire	Madagascar	Senegal	

MIDDLE EAST AND NORTH AFRICA

Algeria	Kuwait	Saudi Arabia	United Arab Emirates
Egypt	Lebanon	Sudan	Yemen
Iran, Islamic Rep. of	Libyan Arab Jamahiriya	Syrian Arab Rep.	
Iraq	Morocco	Tunisia	
Jordan	Oman	Turkey	

SOUTH ASIA

Afghanistan	Bhutan	Nepal	Sri Lanka
Bangladesh	India	Pakistan	

EAST ASIA AND PACIFIC

Cambodia	Korea, Dem. Peo. Rep.	Mongolia	Singapore
China	Korea, Rep. of	Myanmar	Thailand
Hong Kong	Lao Peo. Dem. Rep.	Papua New Guinea	Viet Nam
Indonesia	Malaysia	Philippines	

LATIN AMERICA AND CARIBBEAN

Argentina	Cuba	Honduras	Peru
Bolivia	Dominican Rep.	Jamaica	Trinidad and Tobago
Brazil	Ecuador	Mexico	Uruguay
Chile	El Salvador	Nicaragua	Venezuela
Colombia	Guatemala	Panama	
Costa Rica	Haiti	Paraguay	

FORMER USSR

Armenia	Georgia	Lithuania	Turkmenistan
Azerbaijan	Kazakhstan	Moldova	Ukraine
Belarus	Kyrgyzstan	Russian Federation	Uzbekistan
Estonia	Latvia	Tajikistan	

INDUSTRIALIZED COUNTRIES

Albania	Finland	Japan	Spain
Australia	France	Netherlands	Sweden
Austria	Germany	New Zealand	Switzerland
Belgium	Greece	Norway	United Kingdom
Bulgaria	Hungary	Poland	United States
Canada	Ireland	Portugal	Yugoslavia (former)
Czech Rep.	Israel	Romania	
Denmark	Italy	Slovakia	

DEVELOPING COUNTRIES

Afghanistan	Egypt	Liberia	Rwanda
Algeria	El Salvador	Libyan Arab Jamahiriya	Saudi Arabia
Angola	Eritrea	Madagascar	Senegal
Argentina	Ethiopia	Malawi	Sierra Leone
Bangladesh	Gabon	Malaysia	Singapore
Benin	Ghana	Mali	Somalia
Bhutan	Guatemala	Mauritania	South Africa
Bolivia	Guinea	Mauritius	Sri Lanka
Botswana	Guinea-Bissau	Mexico	Sudan
Brazil	Haiti	Mongolia	Syrian Arab Rep.
Burkina Faso	Honduras	Morocco	Tanzania, U. Rep. of
Burundi	Hong Kong	Mozambique	Thailand
Cambodia	India	Myanmar	Togo
Cameroon	Indonesia	Namibia	Trinidad and Tobago
Central African Rep.	Iran, Islamic Rep. of	Nepal	Tunisia
Chad	Iraq	Nicaragua	Turkey
Chile	Jamaica	Niger	Uganda
China	Jordan	Nigeria	United Arab Emirates
Colombia	Kenya	Oman	Uruguay
Congo	Korea, Dem. Peo. Rep.	Pakistan	Venezuela
Costa Rica	Korea, Rep. of	Panama	Viet Nam
Côte d'Ivoire	Kuwait	Papua New Guinea	Yemen
Cuba	Lao Peo. Dem. Rep.	Paraguay	Zaire
Dominican Rep.	Lebanon	Peru	Zambia
Ecuador	Lesotho	Philippines	Zimbabwe

LEAST DEVELOPED COUNTRIES

Afghanistan	Chad	Malawi	Somalia
Bangladesh	Ethiopia	Mali	Sudan
Benin	Guinea	Mauritania	Tanzania, U. Rep. of
Bhutan	Guinea-Bissau	Mozambique	Togo
Botswana	Haiti	Myanmar	Uganda
Burkina Faso	Lao Peo. Dem. Rep.	Nepal	Yemen
Burundi	Lesotho	Niger	Zaire
Cambodia	Liberia	Rwanda	Zambia
Central African Rep.	Madagascar	Sierra Leone	

DEFINITIONS

Under-five mortality rate
Number of deaths of children under five years of age per 1,000 live births. More specifically this is the probability of dying between birth and exactly five years of age.

Infant mortality rate
Number of deaths of infants under one year of age per 1,000 live births. More specifically this is the probability of dying between birth and exactly one year of age.

GNP
Gross national product, expressed in current United States dollars. GNP per capita growth rates are average annual growth rates that have been computed by fitting trend lines to the logarithmic values of GNP per capita at constant market prices for each year of the time period.

Life expectancy at birth
The number of years newborn children would live if subject to the mortality risks prevailing for the cross-section of population at the time of their birth.

Adult literacy rate
Percentage of persons aged 15 and over who can read and write.

Primary and secondary enrolment ratios
The gross enrolment ratio is the total number of children enrolled in a schooling level — whether or not they belong in the relevant age group for that level — expressed as a percentage of the total number of children in the relevant age group for that level. The net enrolment ratio is the total number of children enrolled in a schooling level who belong in the relevant age group, expressed as a percentage of the total number in that age group.

Income share
Percentage of private income received by the highest 20% and lowest 40% of households.

Low birth weight
Less than 2,500 grammes.

Underweight
Moderate and severe – below minus two standard deviations from median weight for age of reference population;
severe – below minus three standard deviations from median weight for age of reference population.

Wasting
Moderate and severe – below minus two standard deviations from median weight for height of reference population.

Stunting
Moderate and severe – below minus two standard deviations from median height for age of reference population.

Total goitre rate
Percentage of children aged 6-11 with palpable or visible goitre. This is an indicator of iodine deficiency, which causes brain damage and mental retardation.

Access to health services
Percentage of the population that can reach appropriate local health services by the local means of transport in no more than one hour.

DPT
Diphtheria, pertussis (whooping cough) and tetanus.

ORT use
Percentage of all cases of diarrhoea in children under five years of age treated with oral rehydration salts or an appropriate household solution.

Children reaching grade 5 of primary school
Percentage of the children entering the first grade of primary school who eventually reach grade 5.

Crude death rate
Annual number of deaths per 1,000 population.

Crude birth rate
Annual number of births per 1,000 population.

Total fertility rate
The number of children that would be born per woman if she were to live to the end of her child-bearing years and bear children at each age in accordance with prevailing age-specific fertility rates.

Urban population
Percentage of population living in urban areas as defined according to the national definition used in the most recent population census.

Absolute poverty level
The income level below which a minimum nutritionally adequate diet plus essential non-food requirements is not affordable.

ODA
Official development assistance.

Debt service
The sum of interest payments and repayments of principal on external public and publicly guaranteed long-term debts.

Contraceptive prevalence
Percentage of married women aged 15-49 currently using contraception.

Births attended
Percentage of births attended by physicians, nurses, midwives, trained primary health care workers or trained traditional birth attendants.

Maternal mortality rate
Number of deaths of women from pregnancy-related causes per 100,000 live births.

MAIN SOURCES

Under-five and infant mortality
United Nations Population Division, UNICEF, United Nations Statistical Division, World Bank and US Bureau of the Census.

Total population
United Nations Population Division.

Births
United Nations Population Division, United Nations Statistical Division and World Bank.

Under-five deaths
UNICEF.

GNP per capita
World Bank.

Life expectancy
United Nations Population Division.

Adult literacy
United Nations Educational, Scientific and Cultural Organization (UNESCO).

School enrolment and reaching grade 5
United Nations Educational, Scientific and Cultural Organization (UNESCO).

Household income
World Bank.

Low birth weight
World Health Organization (WHO).

Breastfeeding
Demographic and Health Surveys (Institute for Resource Development), and World Health Organization (WHO).

Underweight, wasting and stunting
World Health Organization (WHO), and Demographic and Health Surveys.

Goitre rate
World Health Organization (WHO).

Calorie intake
Food and Agriculture Organization of the United Nations (FAO).

Household expenditure on food
World Bank.

Access to drinking water and sanitation facilities
World Health Organization (WHO) and UNICEF.

Access to health services
UNICEF.

Immunization
World Health Organization (WHO) and UNICEF.

ORT use
World Health Organization (WHO).

Radio and television
United Nations Educational, Scientific and Cultural Organization (UNESCO).

Child population
United Nations Population Division.

Crude death and birth rates
United Nations Population Division.

Fertility
United Nations Population Division.

Urban population
United Nations Population Division and World Bank.

Inflation and absolute poverty level
World Bank.

Expenditure on health, education and defence
International Monetary Fund (IMF).

ODA
Organisation for Economic Co-operation and Development (OECD).

Debt service
World Bank.

Contraceptive prevalence
United Nations Population Division, Rockefeller Foundation and Demographic and Health Surveys.

Births attended
World Health Organization (WHO).

Maternal mortality
World Health Organization (WHO).

UNICEF Headquarters
UNICEF House, 3 UN Plaza, New York,
NY 10017, USA

UNICEF Geneva Office
Palais des Nations, CH-1211 Geneva 10,
Switzerland

UNICEF Regional Office for Eastern and
Southern Africa
P.O. Box 44145, Nairobi, Kenya

UNICEF Regional Office for West and
Central Africa
P.O. Box 443, Abidjan 04, Côte d'Ivoire

UNICEF Regional Office for Latin America
and the Caribbean
Apartado Aéreo 7555, Santa Fé de Bogotá,
Colombia

UNICEF Regional Office for East Asia and
the Pacific
P.O. Box 2-154, Bangkok 10200, Thailand

UNICEF Regional Office for the Middle
East and North Africa
P.O. Box 811721, Amman, Jordan

UNICEF Regional Office for South Asia
P.O. Box 5815, Lekhnath Marg,
Kathmandu, Nepal

UNICEF Office for Australia and New
Zealand
P.O. Box Q143, Queen Victoria Building,
Sydney, N.S.W. 2000, Australia

UNICEF Office for Japan
8th floor, United Nations Headquarters
Building, 53-70, Jingumae 5-chome,
Shibuya-ku, Tokyo 150, Japan